Color Atlas of Periodontology

Copyright © J.D. Strahan and I.M. Waite, 1978
This book is copyrighted in England and may not
be reproduced by any means in whole or part.
Distributed in Continental North, South and Central America,
Hawaii, Puerto Rico and the Philippines by
Year Book Medical Publishers, Inc.
By arrangement with Wolfe Medical Publications Ltd.
Printed by Smeets-Weert, Holland
Library of Congress Catalog Card Number: 78–13104
International Standard Book Number: 0–8151–8491–3

Other books in this series already published:
Color atlas of General Pathology
Color atlas of Oro-Facial Diseases
Color atlas of Ophthalmological Diagnosis
Color atlas of Renal Diseases
Color atlas of Venereology
Color atlas of Dermatology
Color atlas of Infectious Diseases
Color atlas of Ear, Nose & Throat Diagnosis
Color atlas of Rheumatology
Color atlas of Microbiology
Color atlas of Forensic Pathology
Color atlas of Pediatrics
Color atlas of Histology
Color atlas of General Surgical Diagnosis
Color atlas of Physical Signs in General Medicine
Color atlas of Tropical Medicine & Parasitology
Color atlas of Human Anatomy
Color atlas of Cardiac Pathology
Color atlas of Histological Staining Techniques
Atlas of Cardiology: ECGs and Chest X-Rays
Color atlas of Neuropathology
Color atlas of Oral Anatomy
Color atlas of Oral Medicine
Color atlas of Gynecological Surgery
    (Volumes 1 and 2; Volumes 3-6 in preparation)

Color Atlas of

Periodontology

J. Dermot Strahan

BDS, FDS, RCS(Eng)
Head of Department of Periodontology,
Senior Lecturer, Institute of Dental Surgery,
Consultant Dental Surgeon,
Eastman Dental Hospital, London

Ian M. Waite

PhD, BDS, FDS, RCS(Eng), FDS, RCS(Edin)
Senior Lecturer and Honorary Consultant
University College Hospital Dental School,
London
Formerly
Senior Lecturer and Honorary Consultant
Royal Dental Hospital School of Dental Surgery,
London.

Year Book Medical Publishers, Inc.
35 East Wacker Drive, Chicago, Ill., U.S.A.

Contents

Preface 7

1. *Anatomy of the periodontium* 9
2. *Aetiology and pathology of periodontal disease* 15
3. *Epidemiology of periodontal disease* 23
4. *Factors which influence host response* 26
5. *Gingival enlargements and mucosal lesions* 30
6. *Acute periodontal conditions* 36
7. *The assessment of the periodontal patient* 40
8. *The control of dental plaque* 44
9. *Scaling and polishing* 50
10. *Subgingival curettage* 55
11. *The gingivectomy procedure* 58
12. *The inverse bevel periodontal flap procedure* 63
13. *The treatment of osseous defects* 69
14. *Frenectomy* 78
15. *The gingival graft procedure* 82
16. *The laterally repositioned flap* 88
17. *Occlusion and periodontal disease* 90
18. *Occlusal adjustment* 96
19. *The rôle of splints in periodontal therapy* 102
20. *Periodontics and restorative dentistry* 107

Appendix 1: Aetiology and pathology of periodontal disease 114

2: Periodontal indices 115

3: Periodontal assessment form 116

4: Sequence for the components of treatment 121

5: Management of the surgical patient 122

6: Local analgesia in periodontal therapy 125

7: Instrumentation for periodontal surgery 126

8: Periodontal bone defects 127

9: Periodontal suturing techniques 129

10: Wound healing 131

Bibliography 133

Index 139

Preface

The atlas presents a pictorial synopsis of the basic theory of periodontology together with a practical guide to techniques of treatment. The accompanying text is a brief review, which is backed up by a selective bibliography. The atlas is designed for use by dentists, dental ancillaries and students and it is anticipated that it will serve both as an introduction to periodontics and as an aid to revision.

The authors wish to express gratitude to the following for their contribution of photographs for inclusion in the atlas: Professors W A S Alldritt and I R H Kramer, Drs G C Blake, D E R Cornick and H N Newman, and Messrs A Clark, M B Edwards and K W Lee. Acknowledgement is also due to the following authors of papers who very kindly gave permission for diagrams to be reproduced from their publications: Professors J Lindhe, M Listgarten, H Löe and H R Mühlemann, and Drs G M Bowers, B Ellegaard and J C Greene. These papers were published in the Helvetica Odontologica Acta, International Dental Journal, Journal of Dental Research, Journal of Periodontology, Journal of Periodontal Research and Oral Sciences Review. The authors are grateful to the editors of these publications for their cooperation.

Finally we would like to offer our thanks to Mr James Morgan who has helped with many of the photographs and Miss Nicola Robson who has prepared the typescripts.

One of the authors (J D S) wishes to thank the other (I M W) for the time and skill devoted to the preparation of all the line drawings.

1. Anatomy of the periodontium

The supporting tissues

1. The alveolar bone which provides support for the teeth is made up of the outer cortical plates, trabeculated cancellous bone and the bundle bone of the sockets. The sockets are perforated by the blood vessels supplying the periodontal ligament. These vessels anastomose with others entering the socket near the apex and at the gingival margin.

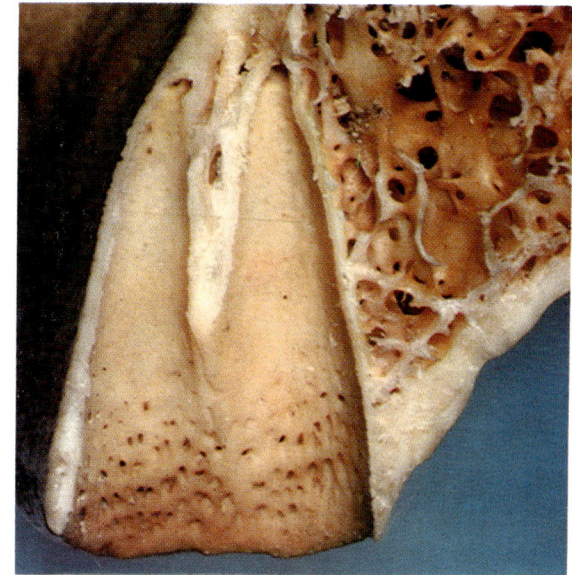

2. The teeth are attached to the sockets by the connective tissue fibres of the periodontal ligament. Most of these fibres run apically in an oblique direction from bone to cementum. However, near the crest of the alveolus and at the apex the main orientation is perpendicular to the root surface. The fibres are embedded in bone and cementum as Sharpey's fibres. The periodontal ligament also contains blood vessels, lymphatics, nerves, and cell rests of Malassez.

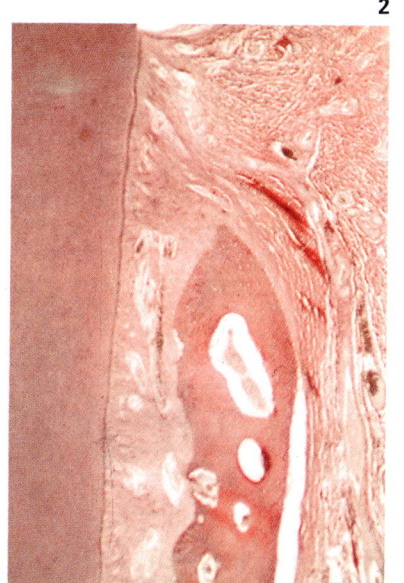

3. Where there are defects in the alveolar bone these can predispose to gingival recession. The regions most frequently involved are the vestibular aspects of the upper and lower canine and lower incisor teeth, and the palatal aspects of upper first molars. The circumscribed defects are called fenestrations and the clefts are called dehiscences.

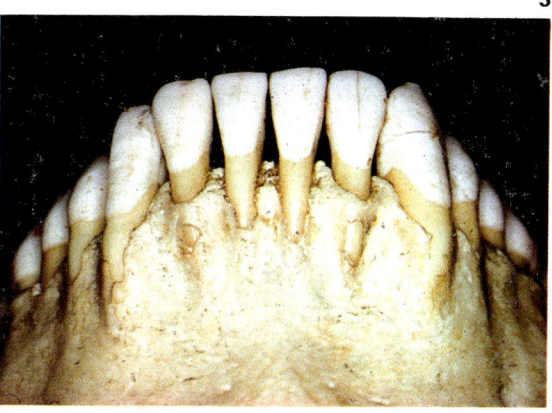

The dento-gingival junction

4. In health there is a gingival sulcus which is about 0.5mm in depth between the tooth and the gingiva; this is lined by unkeratinized epithelium (A). At the base of the gingival sulcus there is the junctional epithelium (B), which is attached to the tooth surface by the basal lamina and hemidesmosomes. The junctional epithelium is relatively weak and is disrupted by probing or other instrumentation. The clinical depth of the gingival sulcus (D) is thus greater than (C) the anatomical depth of sulcus (Listgarten 1972).

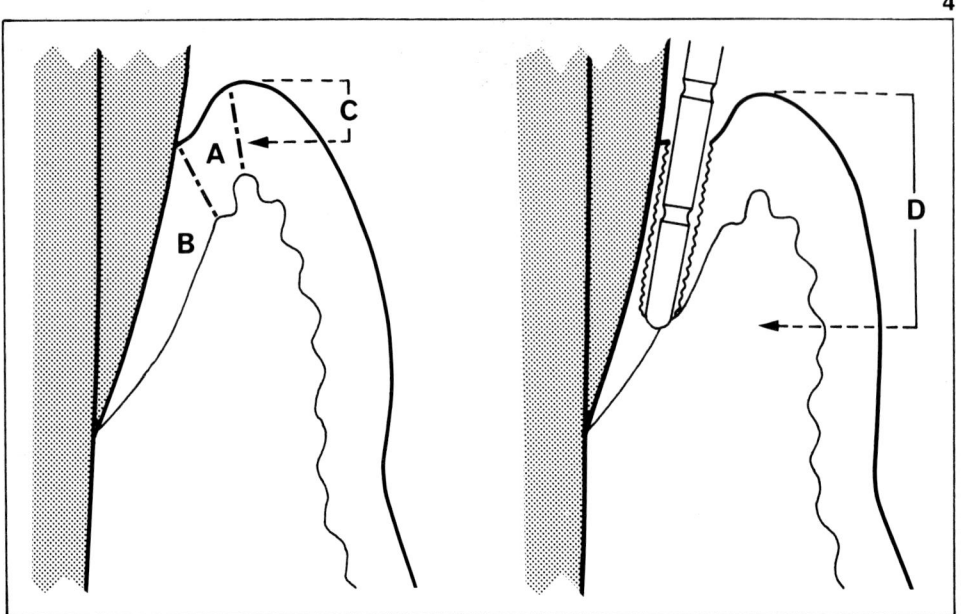

5. The collagen fibres of the gingiva contribute to the adaptation of the soft tissues to the tooth. They are classified as: (A) alveolo-gingival, (B) dento-gingival, (C) transeptal, (D) circular, (E) longitudinal.

These fibre bundles intermingle and anastomose with each other (Melcher and Eastoe 1969).

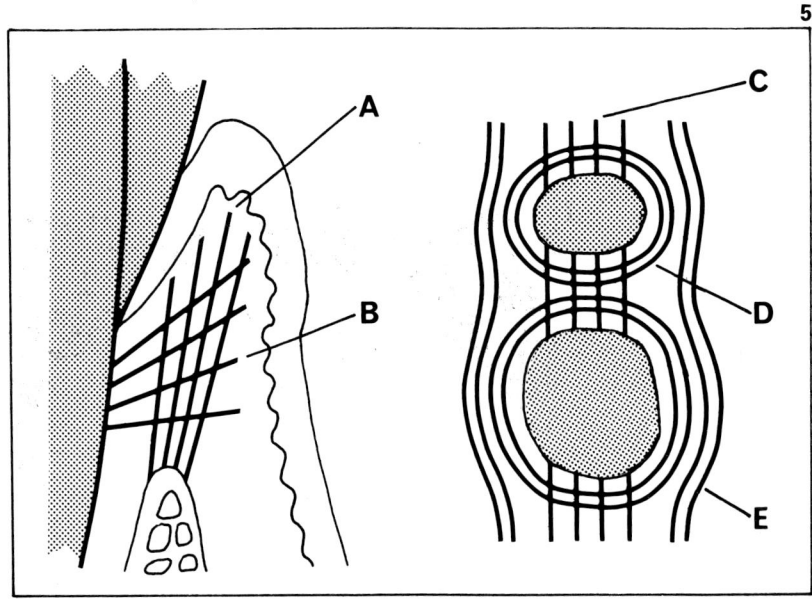

The investing soft tissues

6 & 7. The free gingiva (A) is composed of the interdental papillae (B) and the marginal gingiva (C). A free gingival groove is present in some subjects and this corresponds approximately to the base of the gingival sulcus (Ainamo and Löe 1966). The attached gingiva (D) extends from the level of the base of the gingival sulcus to the muco-gingival junction. The epithelium of the gingiva is keratinized or parakeratinized, and the corium contains dense collagen bundles which firmly attach the gingiva to bone and extra alveolar cementum.

At the muco-gingival junction there is a change to non-keratinized alveolar mucosa (E). This is loosely attached to the periosteum and there are elastic fibres in the corium. The blood supply to the gingiva is derived mainly from the periosteal blood vessels. The interproximal papillae are supplied from capillary loops from the periodontal ligament and also from the crestal bone (Folke and Stallard 1967).

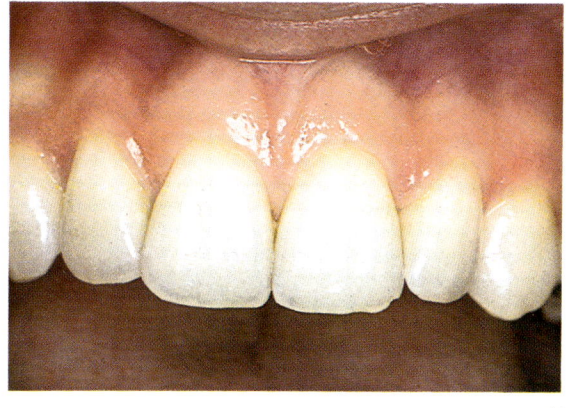

8. The colour of gingiva and mucosa varies between different races. It ranges from pale pink (**6**) to dark brown or black in colour. The pigmentation is often unevenly distributed.

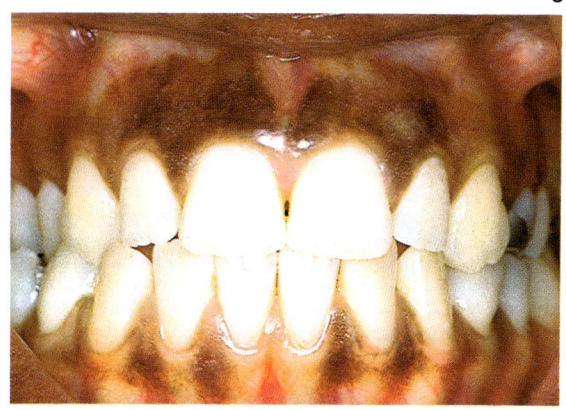

9. The convexity of the crown surface and the tapered margin of the free gingivae promote the deflection of particles over the entrance of the gingival sulcus onto the outer surface of the gingivae.

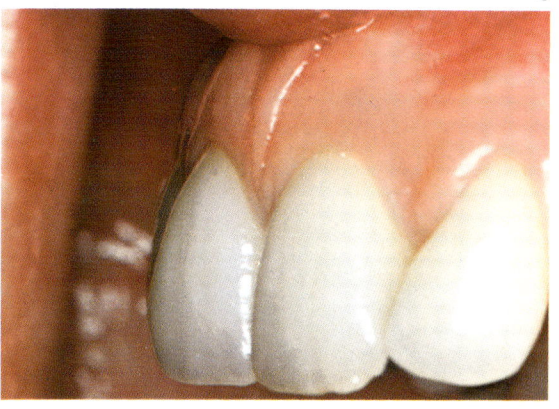

The investing soft tissues

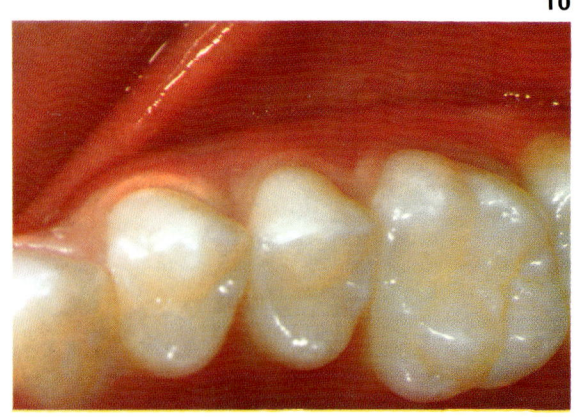

10. The interproximal papillae are protected from trauma during mastication by the contact points and by the marginal ridges of the posterior teeth.

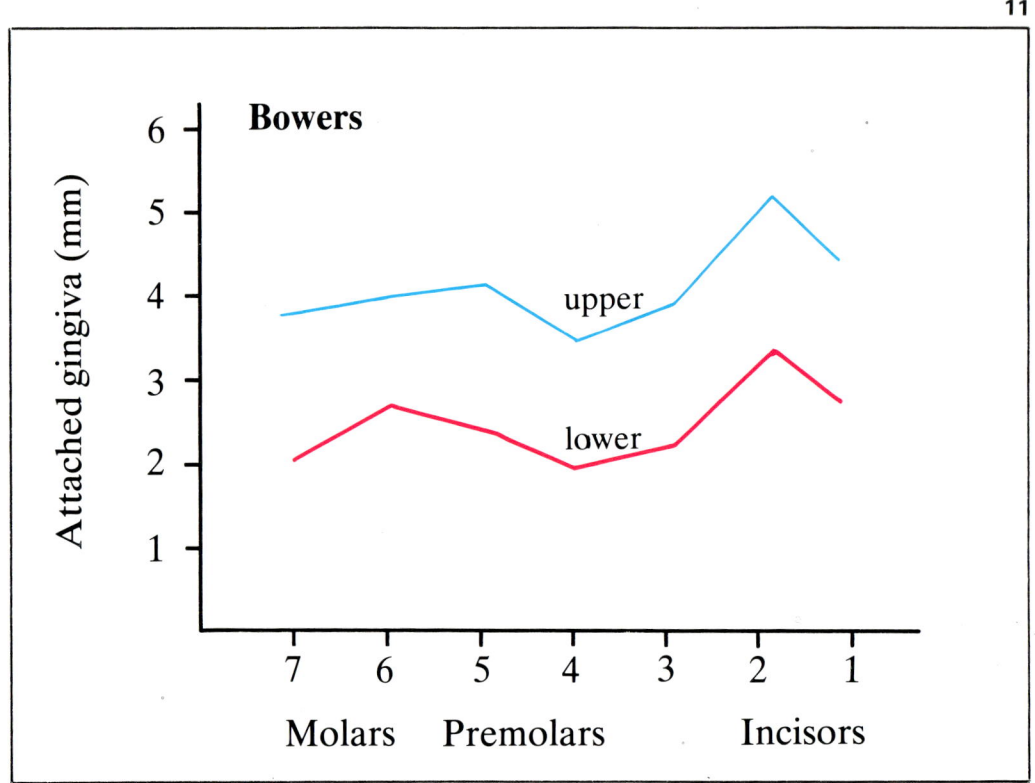

11. The width of the attached gingiva varies between individuals and also depends on the site in the mouth (Bowers 1963). It has been suggested that a width of attached gingiva of at least one millimetre is necessary for gingival health (Lang and Löe 1972), although this has been disputed (Miyasato et al 1977).

The investing soft tissues

12. There are a number of factors which predispose to gingival recession, for example, a labially displaced tooth as in this patient and alveolar bone dehiscence (**3**).

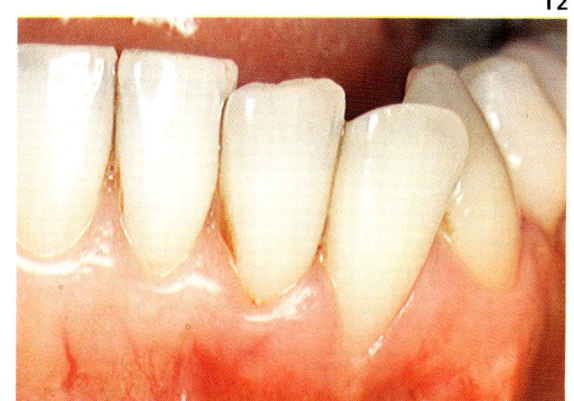

13. Recession is also caused by an increased overbite where there is direct trauma to the gingivae by the opposing teeth.

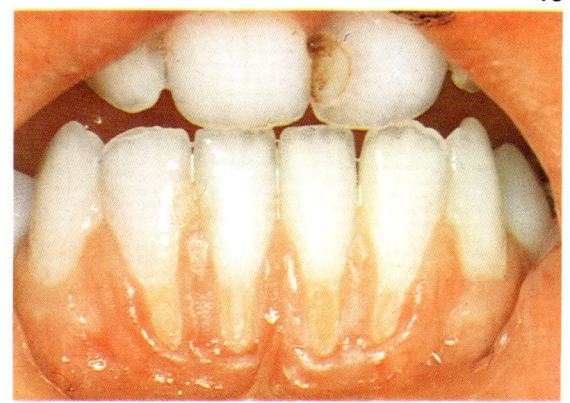

14. A high frenal attachment may result in there being no attached gingivae with consequent displacement of the gingival margin by muscle activity.

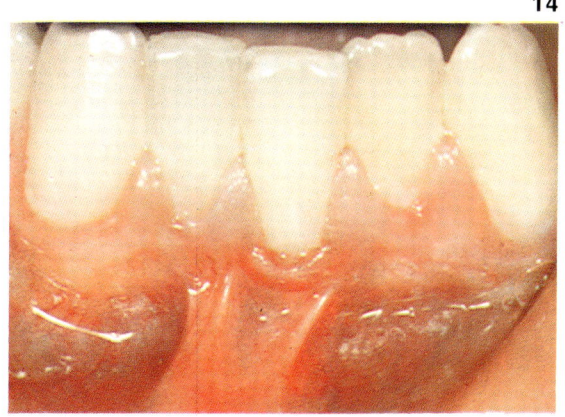

15. The cause of generalised recession is often difficult to diagnose. Possible aetiological factors include chronic periodontal disease, and trauma from incorrect toothbrushing.

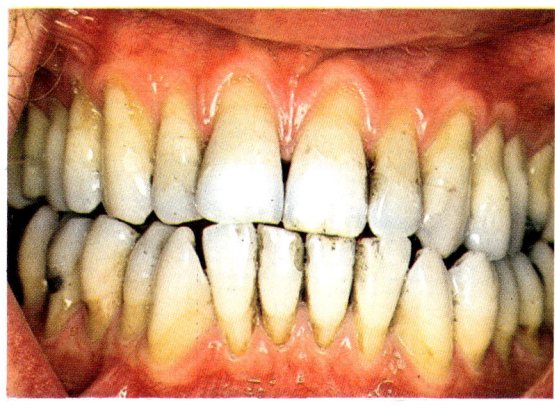

Congenital and developmental abnormalities

16. Fibrous tuberosities are commonly associated with pocketing on the distal and palatal aspects of maxillary third molars. Similar enlargements are sometimes found in the lower retromolar regions. These abnormalities frequently occur bilaterally.

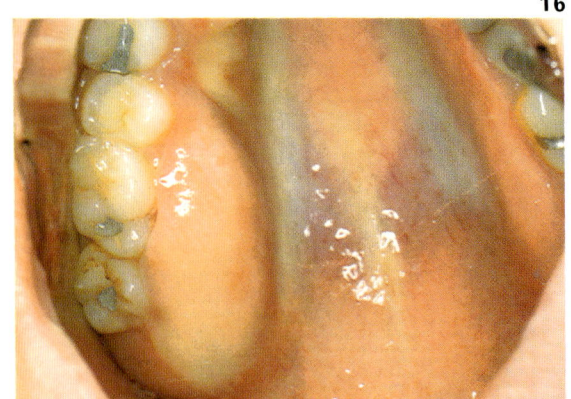

17. Fibromatosis gingivae is a relatively rare condition which may present with the eruption of the primary or secondary dentition or both. The aetiology is obscure and hence the condition has been termed idiopathic hyperplasia. A hereditary basis is supported by the occurrence of the lesion in blood relations.

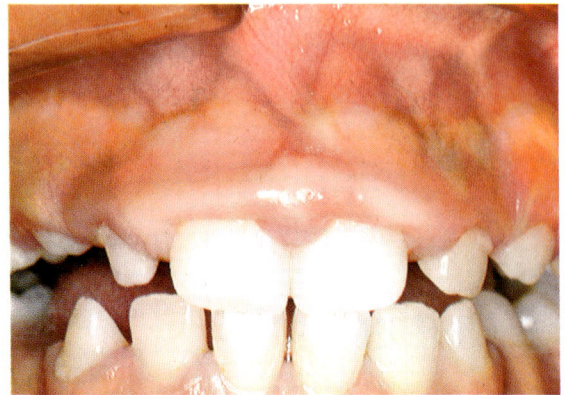

18. A developmental abnormality in tooth form may influence plaque retention and hence cause local exacerbation of periodontal disease. The groove on this tooth has allowed plaque to accumulate and spread up the root surface with resultant localised deep pocket formation.

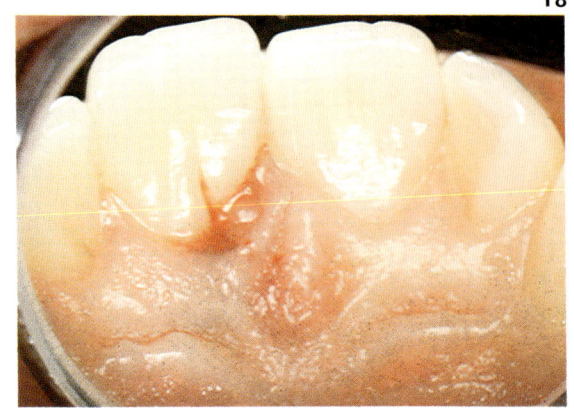

19. The x-ray shows the groove extending to the apical one-third and there is an associated bone defect.

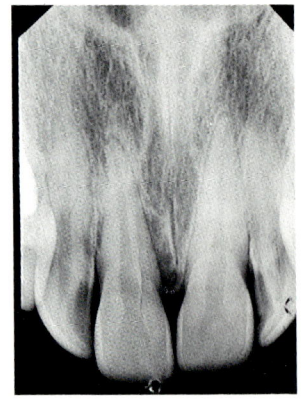

2. Aetiology and pathology of periodontal disease (see Appendix 1)

Tooth deposits

20. A clean tooth surface exposed to the oral environment rapidly accumulates an amorphous protein film called pellicle. This deposition has been attributed to the instability of salivary proteins, and to the surface characteristics of apatite (Jenkins 1970).

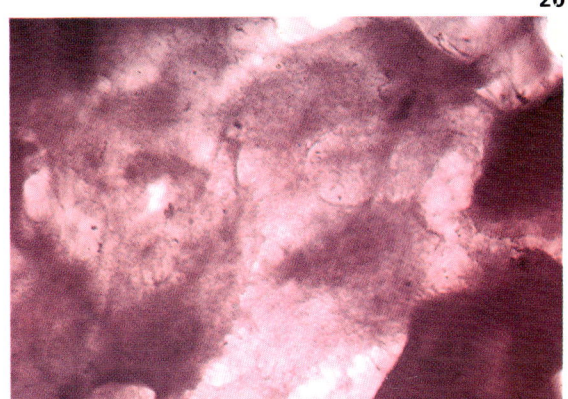

21. The pellicle is soon colonised by bacteria to form plaque. The initial microorganisms are mainly gram positive cocci. Some of these bacteria synthesise extra-cellular polysaccharides, for example dextran, which enable them to adhere to the pellicle and provide resistance to subsequent displacing forces (Gibbons and Van Houte 1973).

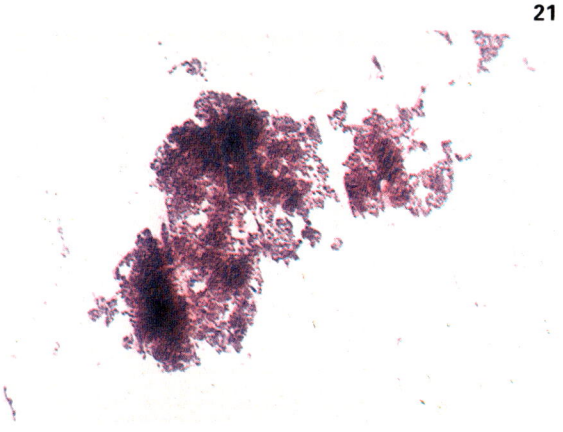

22. In two to four day old plaque, filament and rod-shaped organisms can be seen in greater numbers. As plaque matures there is an increase in the number of gram negative microorganisms. In six to twelve day old plaque, vibrios and spirochaetes become more evident. Desquamated epithelial cells become incorporated in the matrix (Löe, Theilade and Jensen 1965).

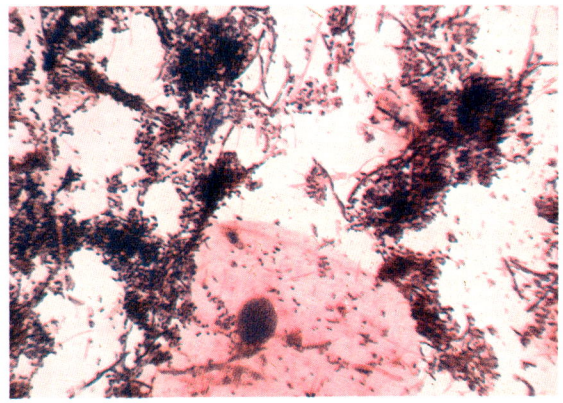

Tooth deposits

23. The scanning electron micrograph shows the complexity of the structure of plaque. Changes in the flora with time may be caused initially by the surface apposition of fusiform, filamentous or other microorganisms on an early plaque composed mainly of cocci. Subsequently, the oxygen tension and the concentration of nutrients within the plaque will determine the relative rate of cell division and hence the ratios of the various microorganisms (Listgarten *et al* 1975). In periodontal pockets where the oxygen tension is low, seventy per cent of the microorganisms are gram negative anaerobic rods (Crawford *et al* 1975).

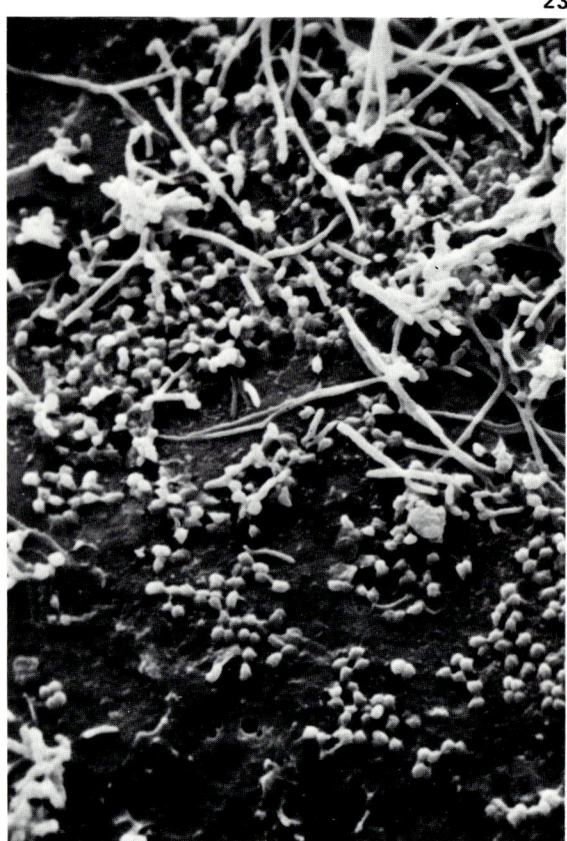

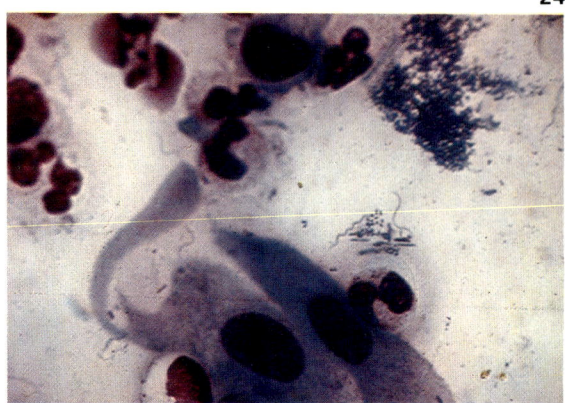

24. A sample of the various cells within the gingival sulcus or the periodontal pocket may be removed on a plastic strip and stained as on this preparation. A variety of bacterial cells can be seen and in response to their presence there has been a migration of leucocytes into the gingival sulcus. Epithelial cells are also evident, these having been released by the turnover of the junctional epithelial cells (Attström 1970).

25. A fluid is released into the gingival sulcus and this may be collected by a variety of techniques, for example on filter paper strips. There is minimal gingival fluid flow from the healthy sulcus, but as inflammation worsens the fluid increases (Löe and Holm-Pedersen 1965). Gingival fluid is formed from serum with modification of the constituents during passage through the tissues, there is a higher potassium ion concentration and lower sodium ion concentration in gingival fluid than in serum. The potassium:sodium ratio increases in patients with periodontitis (Krasse and Egelberg 1962, Bang *et al* 1973). Immunoglobulins and complement components are found in gingival fluid. These contribute to the defence mechanisms of the host.

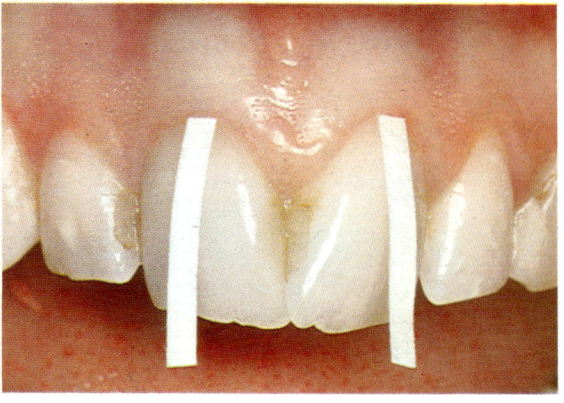

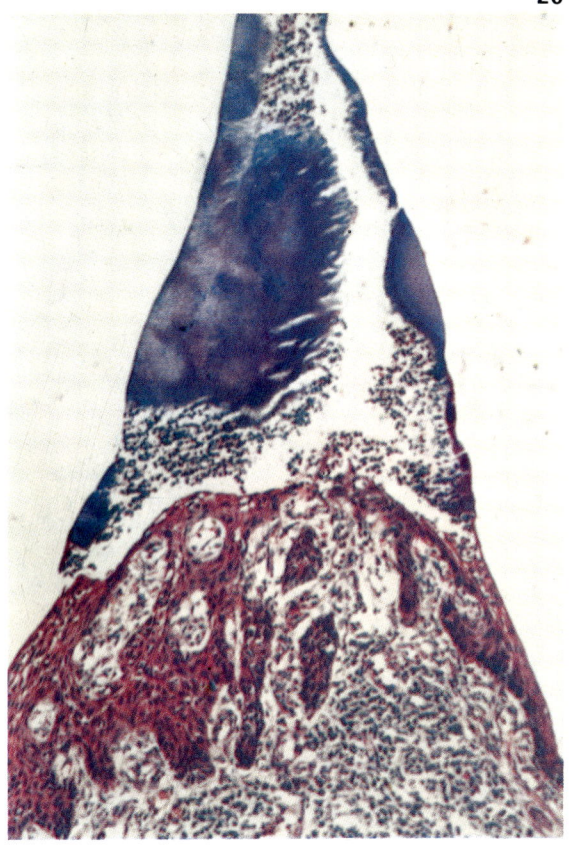

Responses of the tissues

26. The epithelium of the sulcus is in direct contact with sub-gingival plaque. Some of the metabolites from plaque are able to diffuse through the junctional and sulcular epithelium (Schwartz *et al* 1972, Ranney 1970 and Caffesse and Nasjleti 1976). The epithelium is unkeratinized and only a few cell layers in thickness. The permeability is enhanced by inflammation as a result of oedema and changes in the ground substance, which result in separation of the cells and increased diffusion.

27. The metabolites from plaque initiate inflammation and the resultant infiltration by leucocytes can be seen. The tissue reaction is complex and recent research indicates that toxins, enzymes and antigens from plaque may modify and potentiate the inflammation (Simon *et al* 1972, Helderman and Hoogeveen 1976 and Genco *et al* 1974).

28. A variety of methods, including immunofluorescent techniques have been used to detect the presence of immunoglobulins in inflamed periodontal tissues (Mackler *et al* 1977). Fluorescing antibodies can be seen within the plasma cells in this section of gingival tissue. These have probably been produced as a humoural immunological response to plaque antigens. The production of antigen-antibody complexes within the tissues activates complement with the release of biologically active products which have vaso-active properties and are chemotactic to leucocytes. The latter characteristic is contributory to the increase in the number of polymorphonuclear cells in the inflamed tissue.

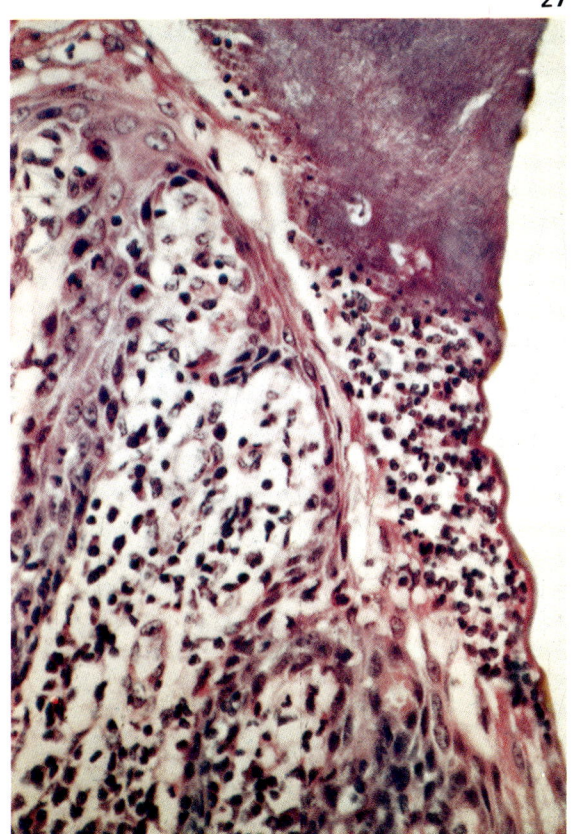

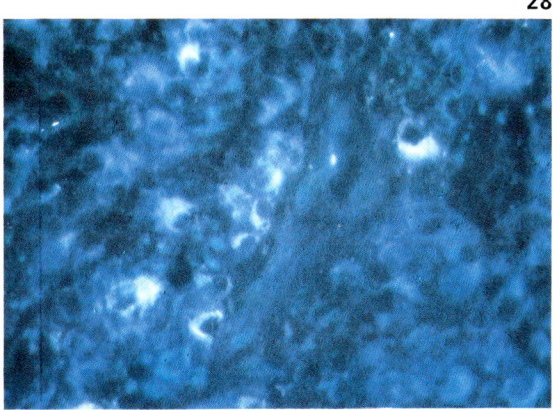

Responses of the tissues

29. The electron micrograph shows lysosomal granules being released from a polymorphonuclear leucocyte. These granules contain enzymes and substances capable of releasing histamine from mast cells. The presence of these substances in the tissues may cause some of the tissue damage in periodontal disease (Taichman 1970).

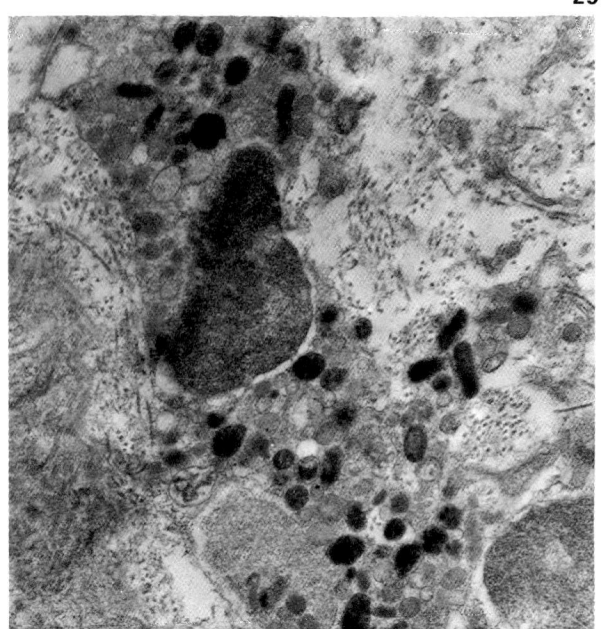

30. Both plasma cells and lymphocytes are evident as components of the inflammatory infiltrate in gingivitis and periodontitis. Correlation has been shown between the degree of periodontal disease and in-vitro lymphocyte transformation (Ivanyi and Lehner 1970, Horton *et al* 1972 and Smith and Lang 1977). These results support the concept that some of the tissue changes in chronic periodontal disease are caused by a cellular immune reaction.

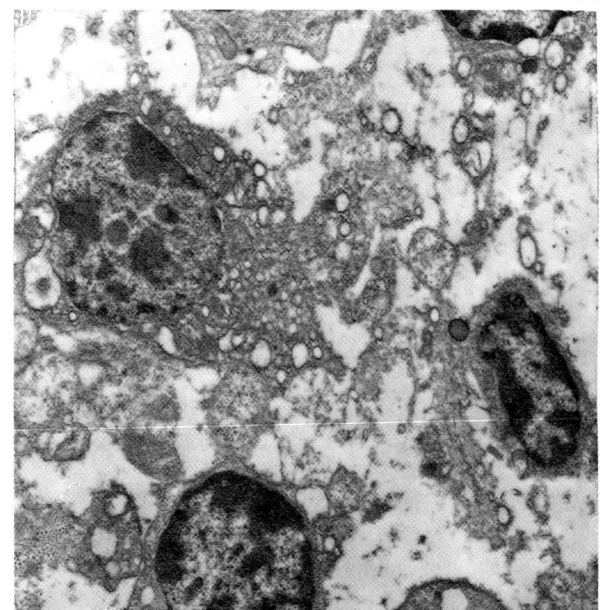

At present the precise mechanisms causing tissue damage in periodontal disease are not known. It seems unlikely that soluble bacterial products directly damage the epithelial cells or connective tissue structures, or that the changes in periodontal disease are solely attributable to an inflammatory response caused by these agents. Antigens from plaque probably initiate inflammation and thereafter the response is sustained by a variety of processes. The factors involved in the disease process probably include immune complexes, complement, sensitised lymphocytes, lymphokines, prostaglandins, histamines, kinins, polymorphonuclear leucocytes, lysosomes and macrophages. Periodontal disease is thus a series of interrelated processes; these vary in their rate of progress at different stages of the disease and according to the environment (Taichman 1974).

The relationship between plaque, inflammation and tissue destruction

31. The inflammatory response may be manifested clinically as enlargement of the gingiva caused by vascular proliferation, oedema and fibrosis. A coronal pocket is thus formed with the base at or coronal to the enamel-cement junction. This is termed gingivitis.

32. In contrast there may be destruction of alveolar bone and periodontal fibres and proliferation of the sulcular epithelium, resulting in radicular pocket formation. This is termed periodontitis. Pockets are frequently caused by a combination of gingival enlargement and periodontal destruction.

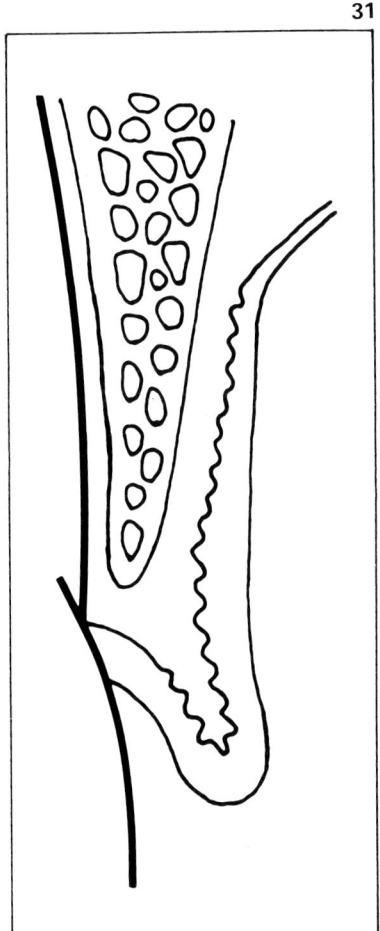
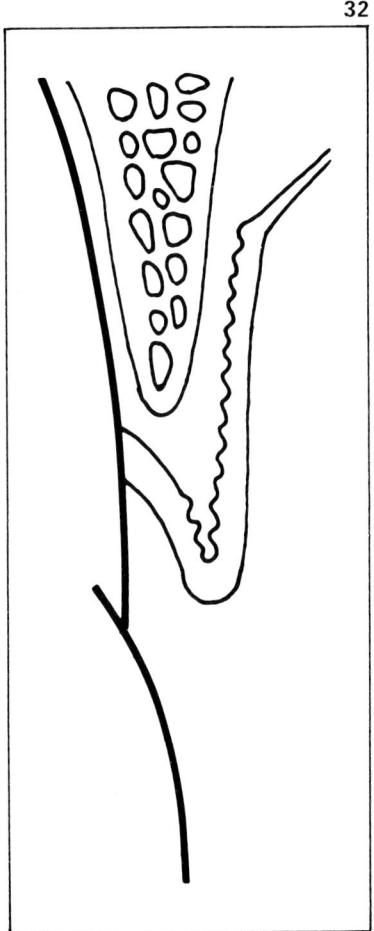

The relationship between plaque, inflammation and tissue destruction

33 & 34. The initiation of gingivitis and periodontitis by plaque deposits has been demonstrated by several workers. For example, Lindhe *et al* (1975) eliminated gingival inflammation in a group of beagle dogs by a treatment regime of twice daily toothbrushing and a weekly prophylaxis.

The group of dogs were then divided into two. The control dogs (indicated by — — — — —) were maintained with zero Plaque Index by twice daily toothbrushing over a four year period. They remained free from gingivitis (**33**) and there was no increase in pocket depth and no loss of periodontal attachment (**34**).

Oral hygiene procedures were withdrawn from some of the dogs with a resultant rapid accumulation of plaque; within a few days these plaque deposits had caused gingival inflammation. Periodontal pockets developed and after about six months there was a progressive loss of periodontal attachment, which amounted to 2.9mm over the four year period.

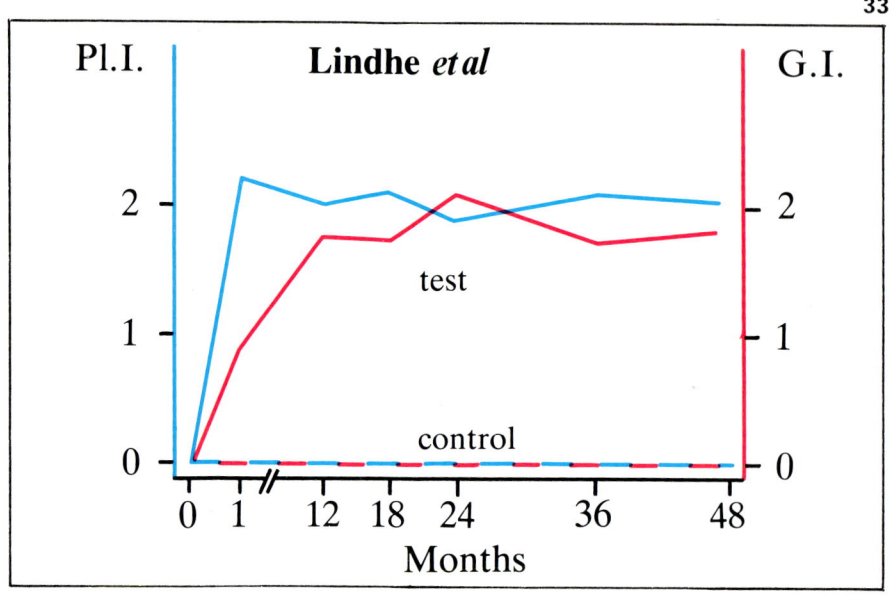

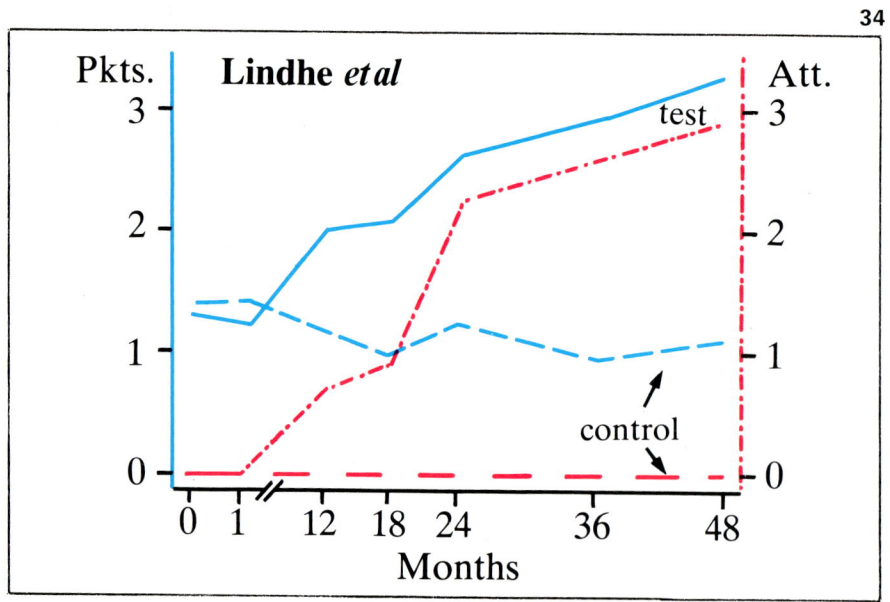

Plaque retaining agents

35. A number of factors can enhance plaque retention and hence contribute to the progression of periodontal disease. The most common of these is calculus. There are a number of theories about how calculus is formed. Calcium and phosphate salts are present in high concentration in saliva and crevicular fluid. Changes in the pH of plaque may be one of the factors causing precipitation. There may be a seeding process involved, and filamentous bacteria have been implicated in the deposition of intracellular and extracellular salts. Supragingival calculus is cream coloured whereas subgingival calculus is brown or black (Jenkins 1970).

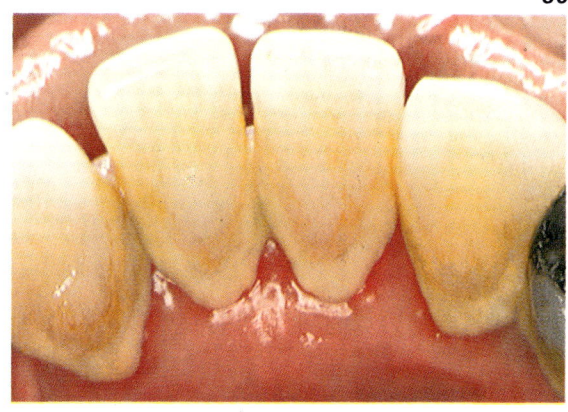

36. Ledges at the cervical margins of amalgam restorations also encourage the accumulation of dental plaque and interfere with its removal. Where ledges are present and particularly if they are located subgingivally, there is a resultant increase in gingivitis and periodontitis (Gilmore and Sheiham 1971).

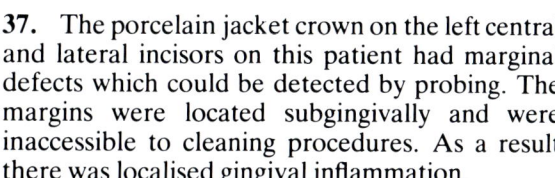

37. The porcelain jacket crown on the left central and lateral incisors on this patient had marginal defects which could be detected by probing. The margins were located subgingivally and were inaccessible to cleaning procedures. As a result there was localised gingival inflammation.

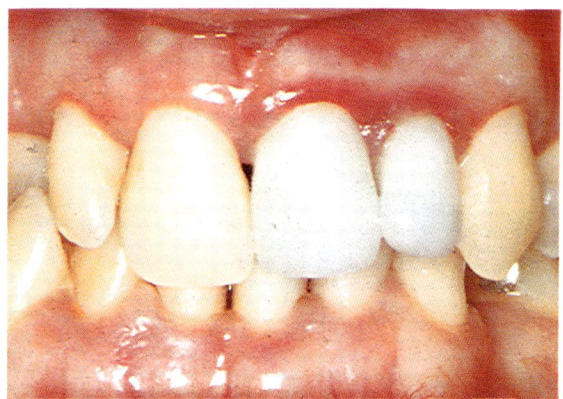

38. Partial denture prostheses may also cause plaque retention with associated periodontal disease and inflammation of the denture bearing area. This damage is minimal provided that good oral hygiene is maintained by the patient and that a satisfactory denture design is used (Bergman *et al* 1971). Orthodontic appliances also increase plaque retention (**254**).

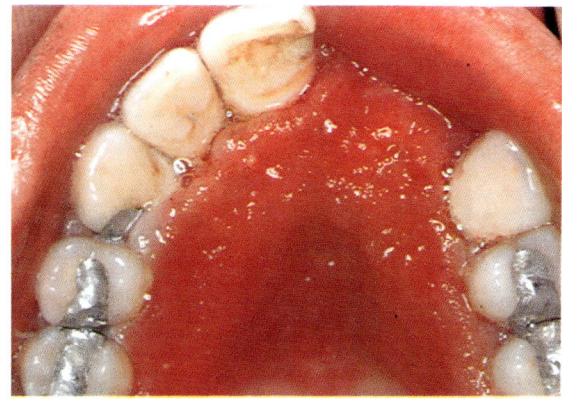

Plaque retaining agents

39. An incompetent lip seal results in drying of the gingiva and hence a reduction in the cleaning action of saliva.

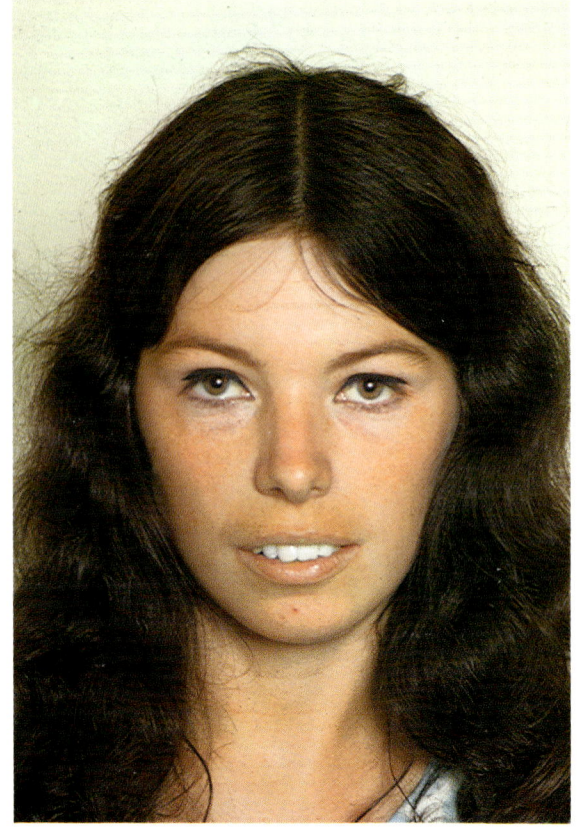

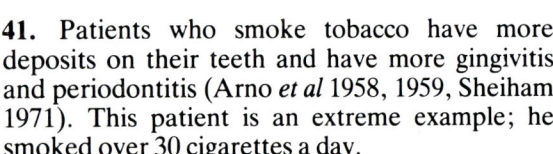

40. There is a resultant increase in gingival inflammation confined to the anterior teeth.

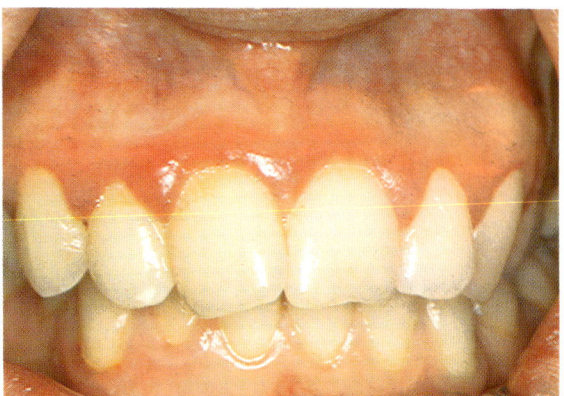

41. Patients who smoke tobacco have more deposits on their teeth and have more gingivitis and periodontitis (Arno *et al* 1958, 1959, Sheiham 1971). This patient is an extreme example; he smoked over 30 cigarettes a day.

There may also be a systemic influence of tobacco smoking on the response of the tissues to plaque. Kenney *et al* (1977) have shown that the polymorphs from the gingiva of smokers were less able to phagocytose particles than those from non-smokers. Smokers are more susceptible to acute necrotising ulcerative gingivitis (**81** and **83**).

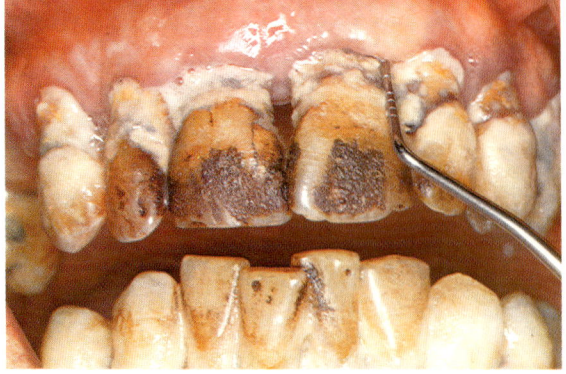

It is concluded that bacterial plaque is the aetiological agent which causes periodontal disease. There are a variety of factors which aid the retention of plaque. The treatment of periodontal disease is based on maintaining the dento-gingival junction free from deposits.

3. Epidemiology of periodontal disease

Introduction

Epidemiology is the quantitative study of the disease status of groups of subjects. Epidemiology may be used to measure the influence of such factors as age, sex, socio-economic status, race and geographic location on periodontal disease. The scope of the present chapter will be to consider this aspect of epidemiology.

The measurement of aetiological agents such as plaque and plaque retaining agents and their influence on periodontal disease is also covered by epidemiology. This aspect of the subject, together with the influence of systemic disorders on the host response to bacteria is covered in Chapters 2 and 4.

The scientific study of the epidemiology of periodontal disease has been made possible by the development of indices. These comprise a series of definitions which enable the status of the periodontium to be measured and provide a method of quantifying the aetiological agents associated with periodontal disease (Appendix 2).

Influence of age and sex

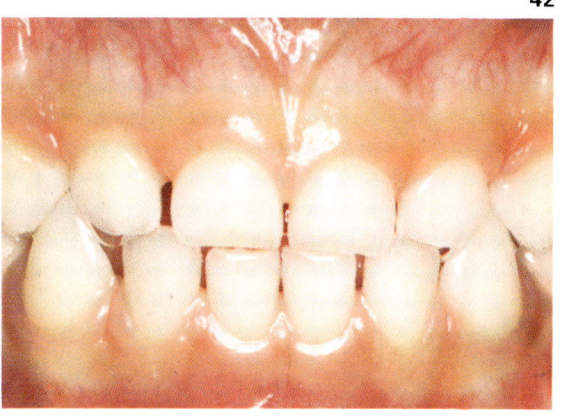

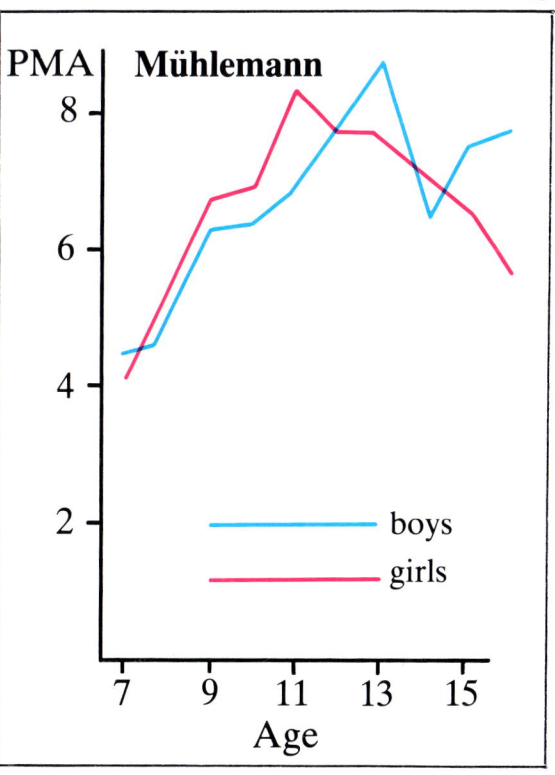

42. Apart from localised inflammation around erupting teeth, periodontal disease is generally not found in very young children even in the presence of abundant plaque deposits (Mackler and Crawford 1973, Cox *et al* 1974). From about the age of five onwards children with inadequate oral hygiene show a progressive increase in gingival inflammation.

43. In the early teens there is a transient sharp rise in gingival inflammation associated with puberty. This occurs earlier in girls than boys. After puberty however girls have less periodontal disease than boys (Mühlemann 1958, Sutcliffe 1972). The trend for there to be less disease in females than in males is also seen in adulthood, and this may be due to the better oral hygiene standards in females.

Influence of age and sex

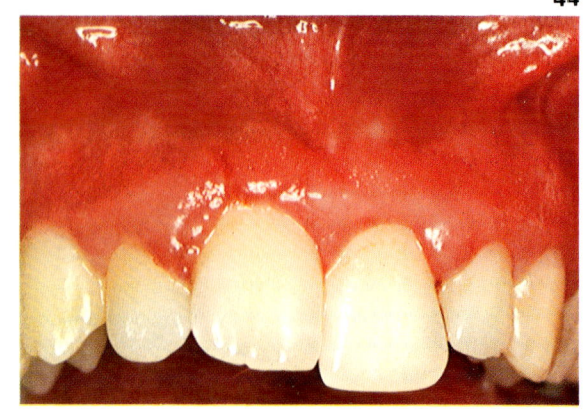

44. Clinical evidence of periodontitis is generally first seen in the mid teens. This 15-year-old boy has gingivitis and also periodontitis with pockets extending beyond the enamel-cement junction on several teeth in the interproximal regions. Lennon and Davies (1974) demonstrated that 46 per cent of 15-year-old children have loss of attachment of at least one millimetre involving one or more teeth.

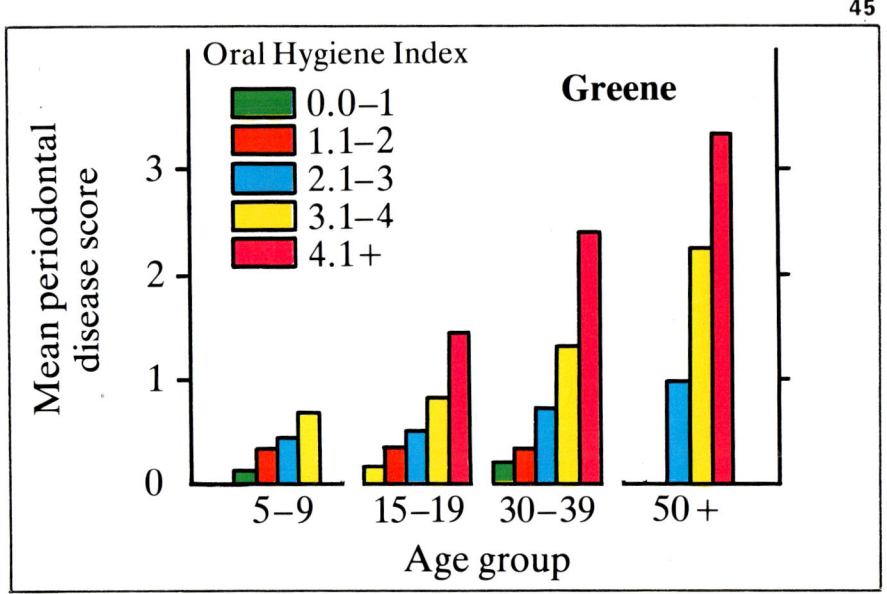

45. During adult life epidemiological studies have shown a progressive increase in periodontal disease with age. However, where good standards of oral hygiene were maintained, periodontitis was not found (Greene and Vermillion 1963). Thus the increase in periodontal disease with age was due to the prolonged exposure of the tissues to plaque metabolites.

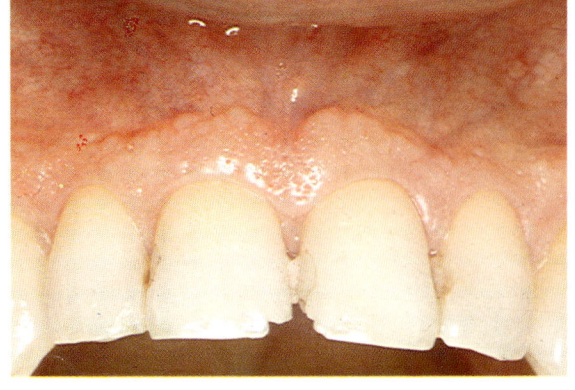

46. The periodontal tissues of older subjects show increased fibrosis, decreased cellularity, and hyalinisation of the periodontal ligament fibres (Grant and Bernick 1972). However, these changes are compatible with health provided plaque control is good. This patient has a healthy periodontium at the age of 68.

Socio-economic factors, geographic distribution and effect of race

47. This study by Greene (1960) shows that there was more periodontal disease in the Indian communities than in the American ones, and also that there was more periodontal disease in the rural areas of India than in the urban areas. This might suggest that social, geographical or racial factors were involved.

48. In the same study Greene related the oral hygiene levels in the Indian and the American communities to the amount of periodontal disease; both groups show a close correlation. Most of the differences can, therefore, be attributed to variation in plaque control rather than to other factors. In some of the developing countries dietary deficiency may be a contributory factor to periodontal disease (Russell *et al* 1965). Russell assessed the correlation between periodontal disease and the concentration in the blood of vitamin A, vitamin C, carotene, thiamine, riboflavin, protein, etc. He also measured the haematocrit, haemoglobin and weight/height ratio. He concluded that none of these factors contributed more than 4 per cent of the variation in Periodontal Index scores between the individuals.

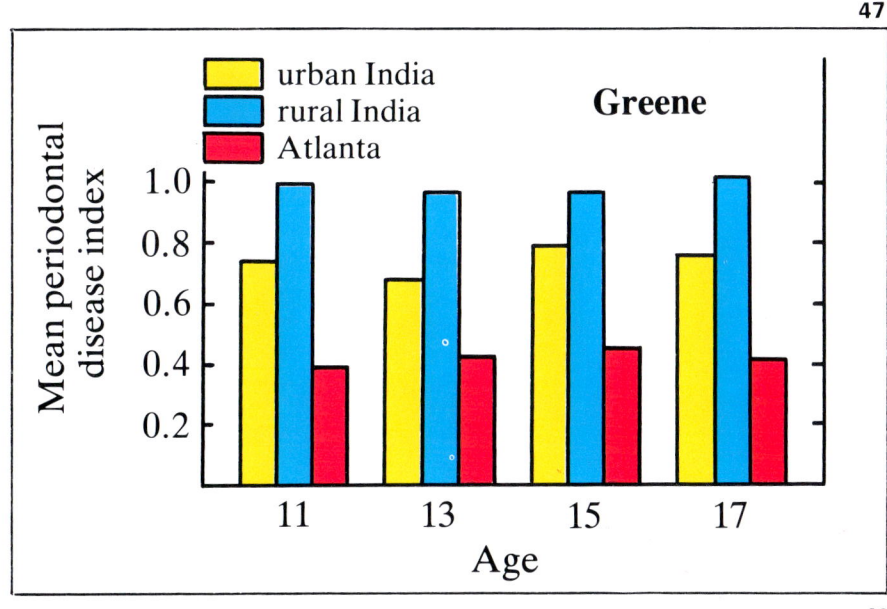

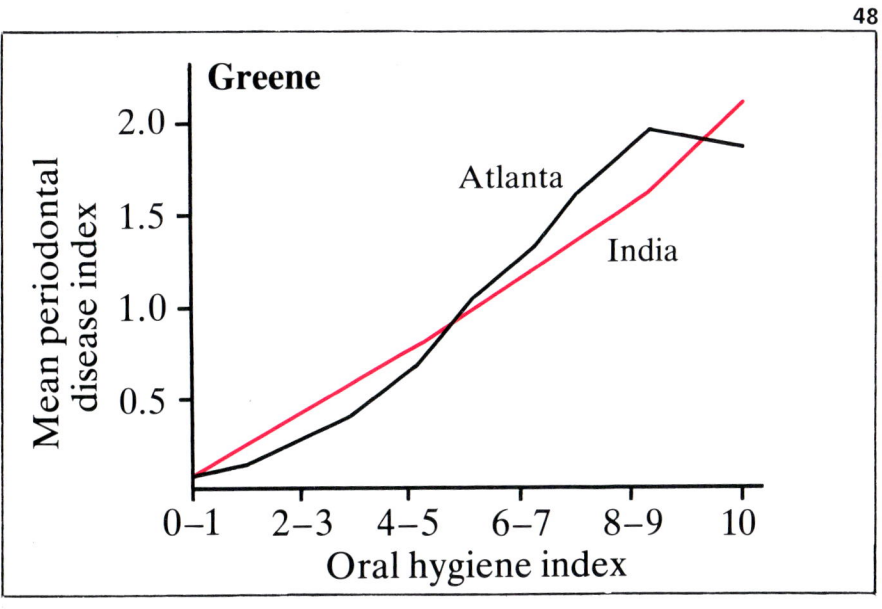

4. Factors which influence host response

Introduction

The response of the periodontal tissues to plaque varies in degree between individuals. This may be caused partly by variation in the local protective mechanisms which are active in the removal of the plaque metabolites (Appendix 1). The inflammatory and immunological reactions to plaque may also differ between subjects. Patients with an enhanced response to plaque need to maintain the highest possible standards of oral hygiene. Priority should be given to these patients particularly in the preliminary stages of treatment when frequent plaque control appointments are indicated. A number of specific systemic factors have been shown to influence the response of the host. The prognosis and choice of a definite treatment plan depends on the nature of any systemic abnormality.

Systemic disease

49. This patient has drug induced agranulocytosis. Blood dyscrasias influence the number and function of the leucocytes and thus alter the resistance of the host. Clinically, there is exaggerated inflammation of the gingiva. Ulceration of the mucosa and abscess formation are common.

Drugs

50. Patients taking hydantoin drugs for epilepsy may develop gross fibrous proliferation of the gingival tissue in response to plaque, with resultant false pocketing. The subsequent retention of increased amounts of plaque in these pockets exacerbates inflammation and hyperplasia. Surgical excision of the hyperplastic tissue often proves necessary for aesthetic or functional reasons. Good oral hygiene has been shown to reduce the proliferation of tissue; however, hyperplasia may gradually recur, necessitating further localised surgery (Donnenfeld *et al* 1974).

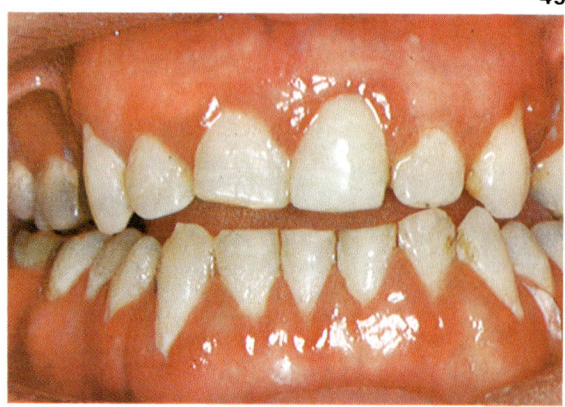

49

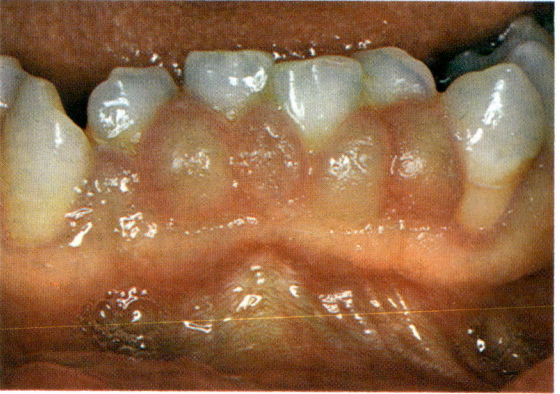

50

Hormonal changes

51. This patient is a diabetic and has severe gingivitis and periodontitis. It has been demonstrated that diabetic patients have more inflammation, and more loss of attachment than non-diabetic patients (Cohen *et al* 1970).

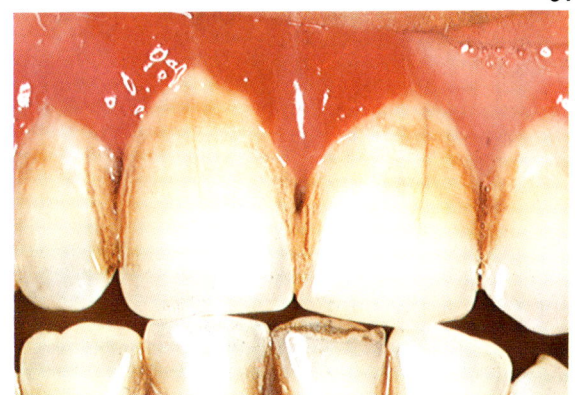

52. At puberty changes in the host response to plaque caused by hormonal factors result in an increase in the degree of gingival inflammation (**43**).

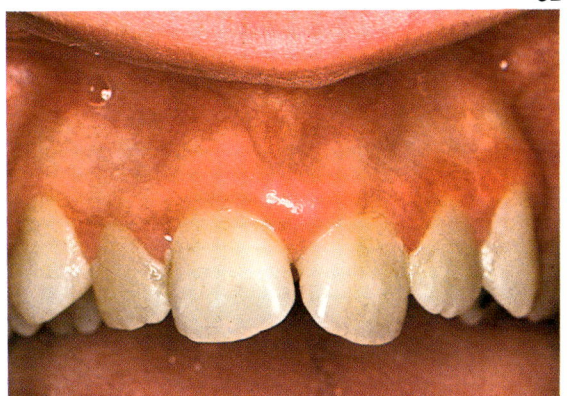

53. The hormonal changes during pregnancy also cause an enhanced host response to plaque (Löe and Silness 1963, Cohen *et al* 1971). Healthy gingivae are not influenced by pregnancy, increased inflammation only occurs when plaque and gingivitis are present initially (Hugoson 1970). The changes are probably caused by raised levels of progesterone which result in increased permeability of the blood vessels and changes in ground substance. The use of oral contraceptives may result in similar but less severe changes in the gingivae (Lindhe and Björn 1967).

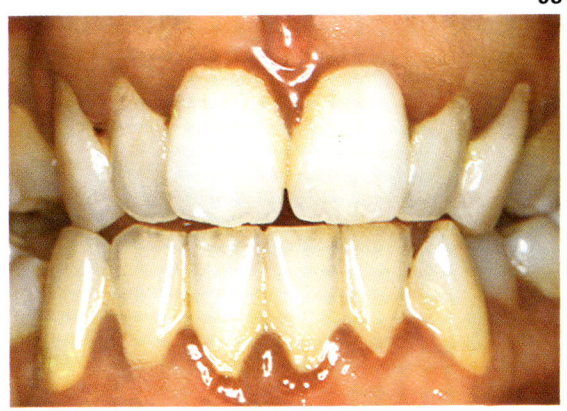

54. After parturition there is resolution of the gingival inflammation to approximately the same level as before pregnancy. Cohen *et al* (1971) have reported that there is no loss of attachment following pregnancy gingivitis. The decision as to whether periodontal surgery is indicated should be made when the improvement in periodontal condition after parturition has occurred.

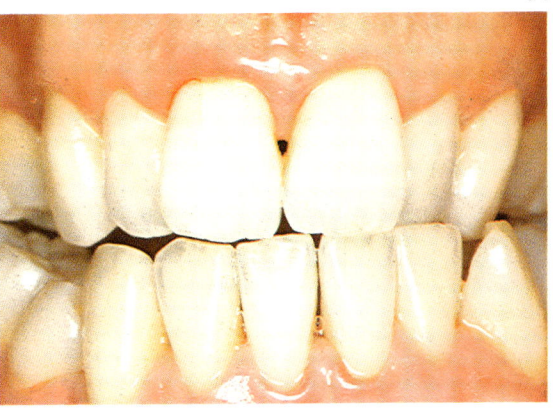

Juvenile periodontitis (periodontosis)

55 & 56. Juvenile periodontitis is an uncommon lesion occurring in late adolescence or young adulthood. Periodontal destruction is usually localised and the teeth most commonly affected are the incisor and first molar teeth.

There may be relatively good oral hygiene and only mild gingivitis in relation to the advanced bone loss. Several factors have been implicated; for example, there may be a genetic abnormality (Baer 1971). Lehner *et al* (1974) report a selective impairment of the cellular immune response to plaque. Patients with B blood group may be more susceptible (Kaslick *et al* 1971) and some studies report a greater incidence in females than males. Treatment is the same as for periodontitis in the adult, that is by plaque control, pocket elimination and extractions where teeth cannot be saved. Provided good oral hygiene is maintained the initial rapid loss of bone can often be arrested.

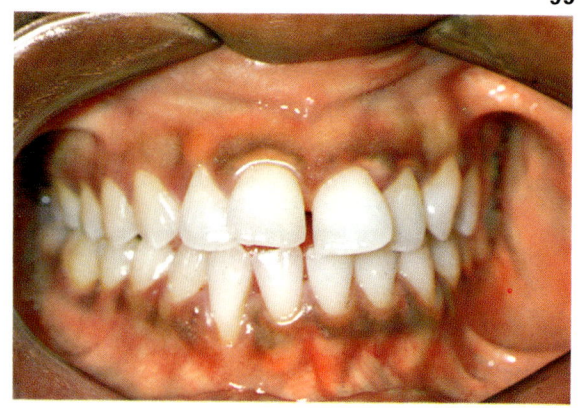

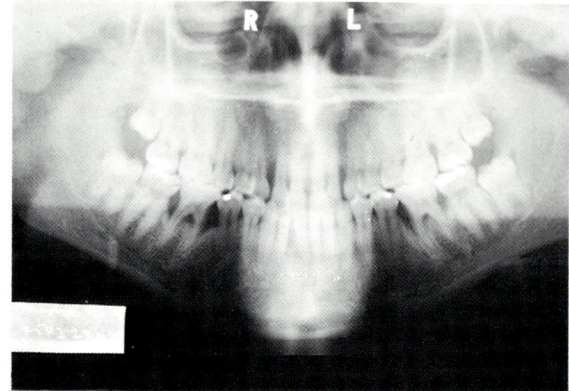

Congenital defects

57. One of the symptoms of the Papillon Lefèvre syndrome is an increased susceptibility to periodontal disease. Gross alveolar bone loss may be found even in the deciduous dentition.

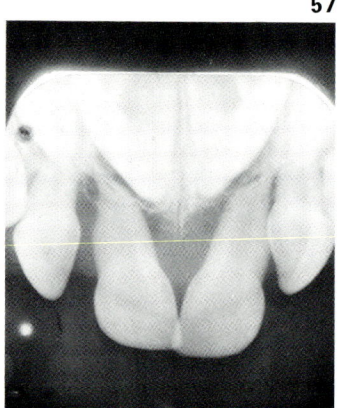

58. The other characteristic feature of the above syndrome is that the epidermis of the palms of the hands and the soles of the feet is thickened.

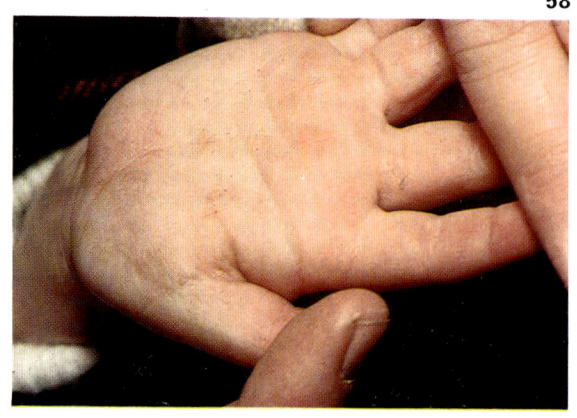

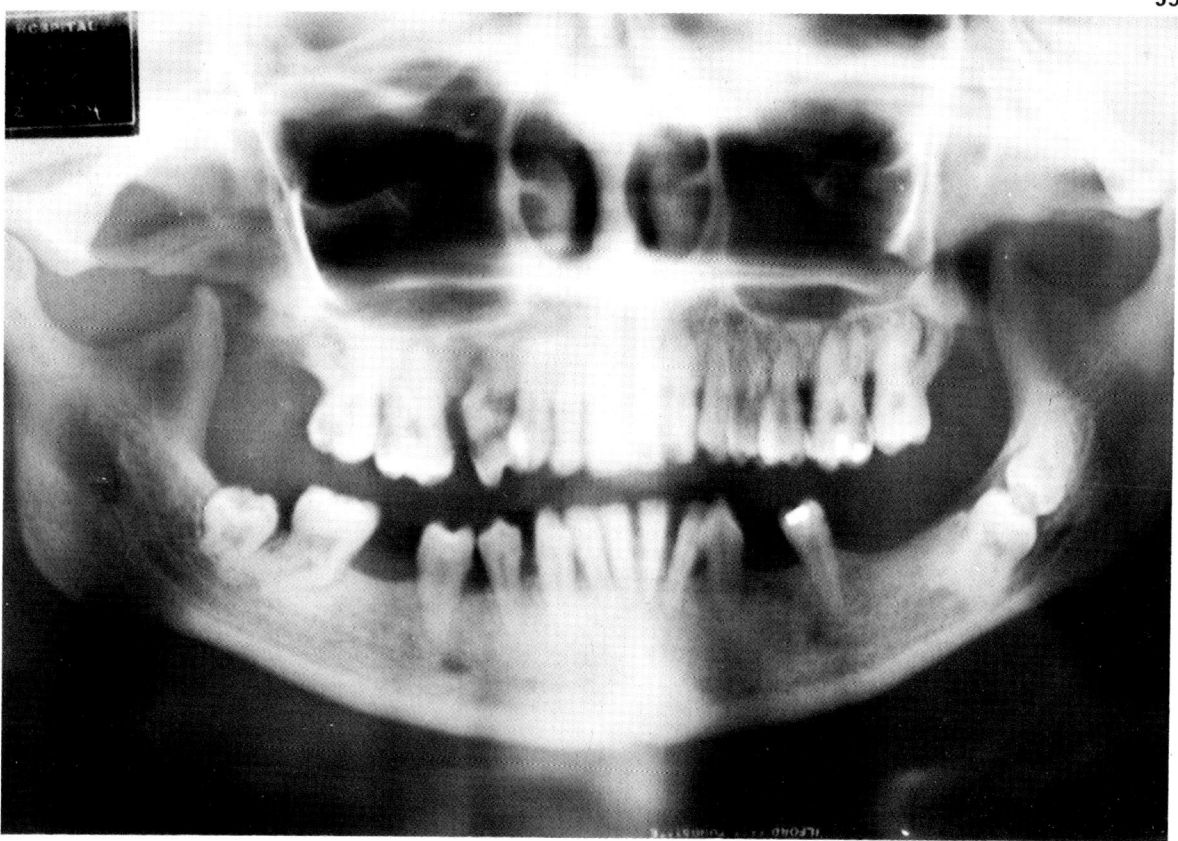

59. Patients with Down's syndrome may have an increased susceptibility to periodontal disease (Saxén *et al* 1977), as well as a number of other oral manifestations including macroglossia, a high arched palate and malformed teeth.

5. Gingival enlargements and mucosal lesions

Gingival enlargements

Generalised gingival enlargement is commonly caused by an inflammatory response to plaque with resultant oedematous hyperplasia (**137**) or fibrous hyperplasia (**146**). There may be systemic factors causing an exaggerated reaction; for example, congenital anomalies (**17**), drug therapy (**50**), or hormonal factors (**52** and **53**). Localised gingival swelling may be due to acute inflammation with abscess formation (**84**). Other relatively common causes of local gingival enlargement are given below. It is important that a diagnosis is made to exclude malignancy.

60. The 'fibrous epulis' is a localised swelling caused by chronic inflammation. There are usually deposits of calculus on the associated teeth which have caused the original irritation. Clinically it is not possible to distinguish it from a fibroma which is less common.

61. Histopathologically the lesion is composed of fibrous tissue at various stages in development with blood vessels and inflammatory cells. There is a covering of stratified squamous epithelium.

62. The pyogenic granuloma arises as a non-specific response to local irritation.

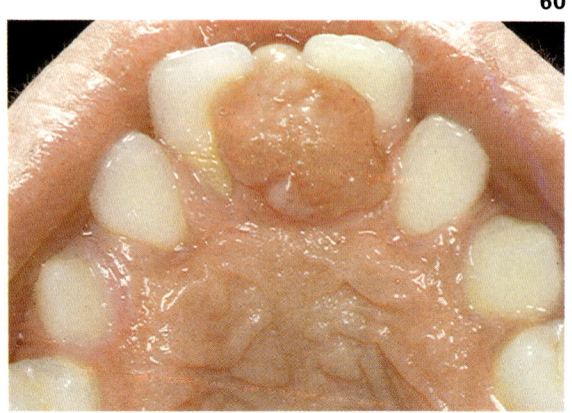

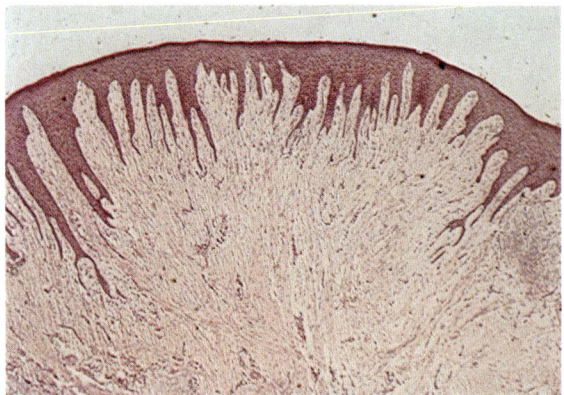

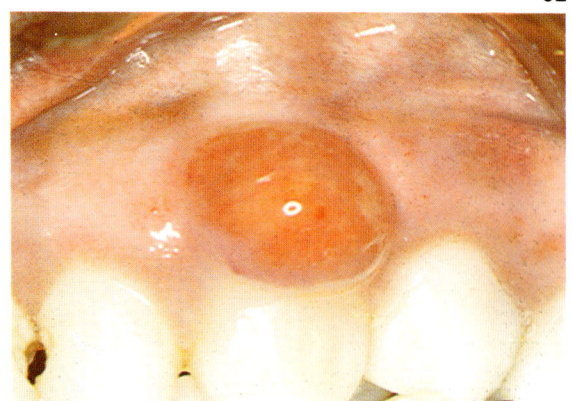

Gingival enlargements

63. It is composed mainly of vascular spaces and fibroblasts. The epithelial surface is thin and if ulceration is present there may be an inflammatory infiltrate.

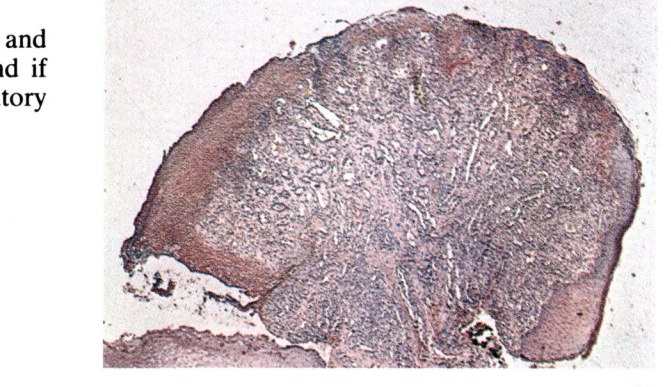

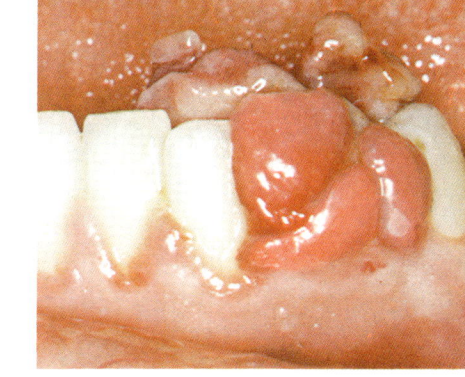

64. The 'pregnancy tumour', which is identical histologically to the pyogenic granuloma, is fairly common and may appear from the third month of pregnancy onwards. It probably represents an intensified response to local minor trauma. This swelling was first noticed by the patient during the sixth month of pregnancy. Surgical excision is indicated during pregnancy if the lesion is causing discomfort or interfering with eating. Removal after pregnancy is preferred as recurrence is less likely. The lesion is treated by excision and the underlying bone is curetted as this reduces the frequency of recurrence. All the deposits must be removed from the teeth.

65. The giant cell granuloma is found on the gingiva or alveolar process. It is often dark red or haemorrhagic in appearance.

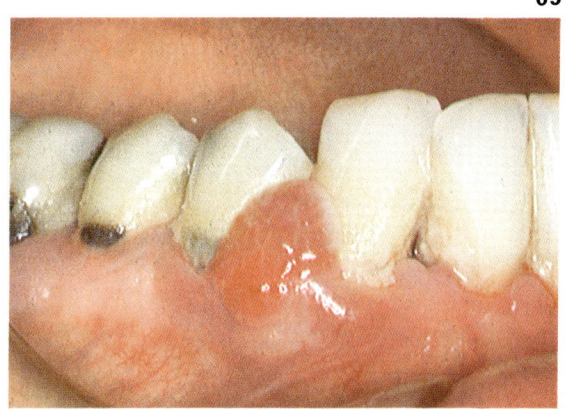

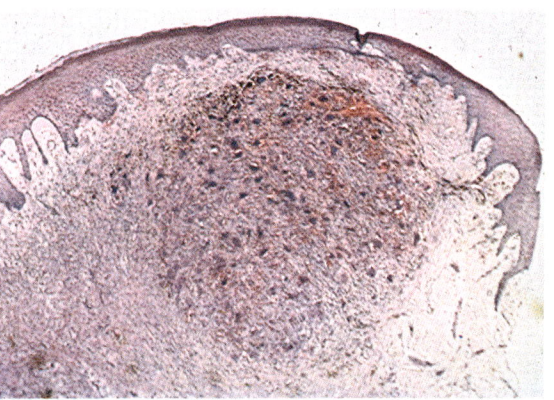

66. Histologically, it consists of a non-encapsulated mass of reticular fibroblasts and multi-nucleated giant cells. There are numerous capillaries. Treatment is by excision and curettage of the base of the lesion. Recurrence is not uncommon, and this is probably because there is no capsule.

Gingival enlargements

67. The papilloma is a relatively common lesion found on the tongue, lips, buccal mucosa, gingiva and palate. It consists of multiple projections comprising thin connective tissue central cores covered with epithelium. Treatment is by excision to include the base of the lesion.

There are many other benign and malignant neoplasms which may involve the gingivae. These are beyond the scope of the present book.

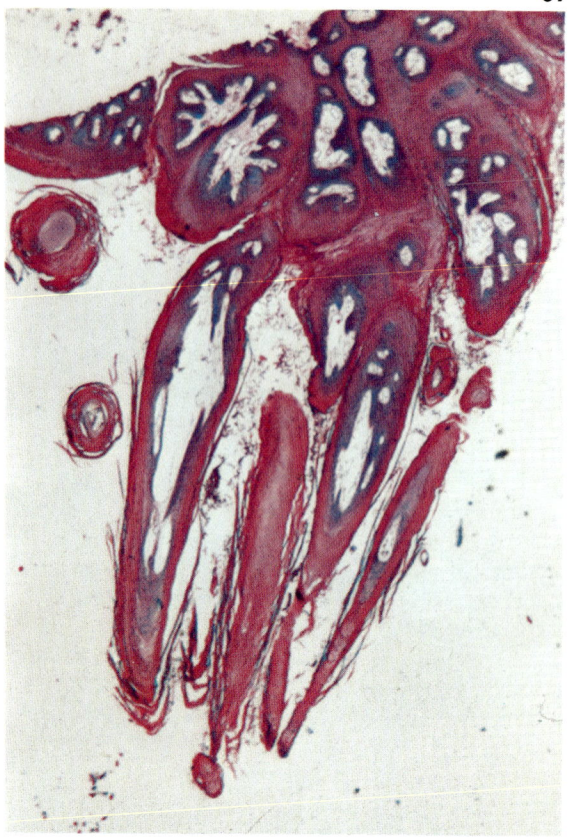

Mucosal lesions

68. Chemical injury to the gingiva and mucosa may result from the use of drugs. This patient has been using a mouthwash containing phenol. A localised lesion may also result from an aspirin tablet retained in the mouth.

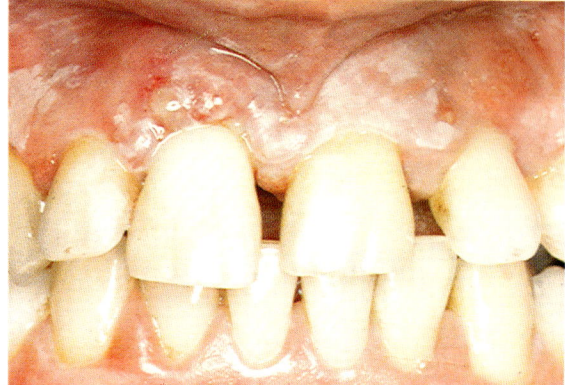

69. Aphthous ulcers occur singly or in groups and appear as round or oval ulcers of varying size. They may be found on the lips, cheeks, tongue, palate, gingivae, floor of mouth or pharynx. They persist for one or two weeks and may recur at varying time intervals. Where the lesions are of longer duration, or a large surface area is involved, symptoms may be reduced by the topical application of a corticosteroid ointment in an adhesive base.

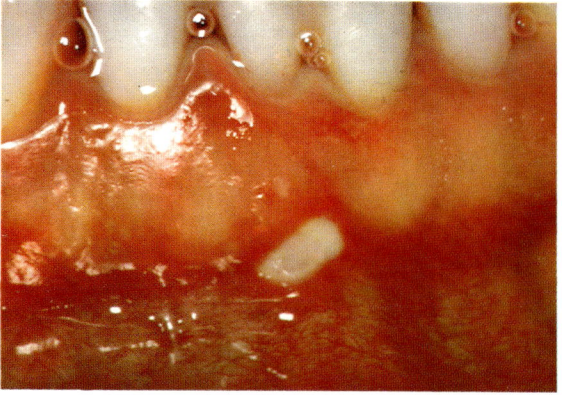

Mucosal lesions

70. Acute herpetic gingivostomatitis caused by the herpes simplex virus is usually preceded by a prodromal sore throat, pyrexia and malaise. Vesicles form on the lips, cheek and tongue, and rapidly rupture to give ulcers.

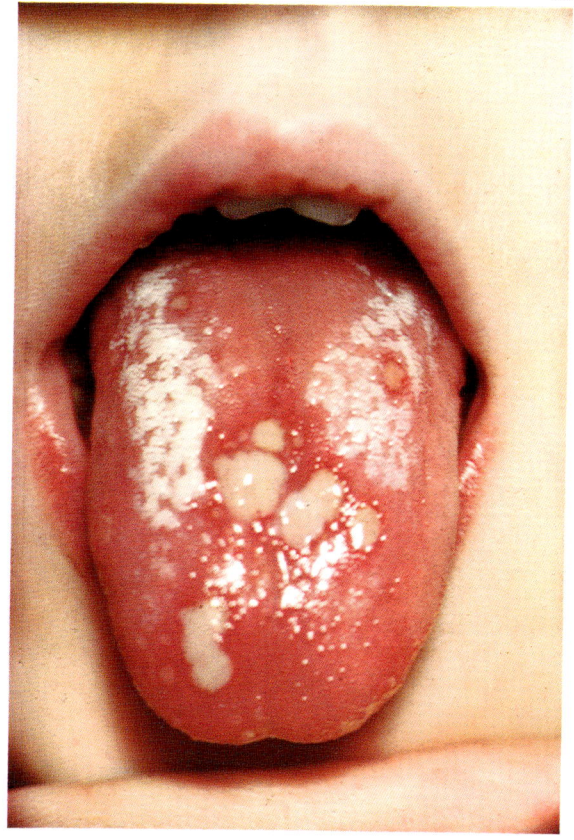

71. The vesicles may also involve the gingivae but these tend to be smaller than elsewhere. The condition is most common in young children but may also affect adults.

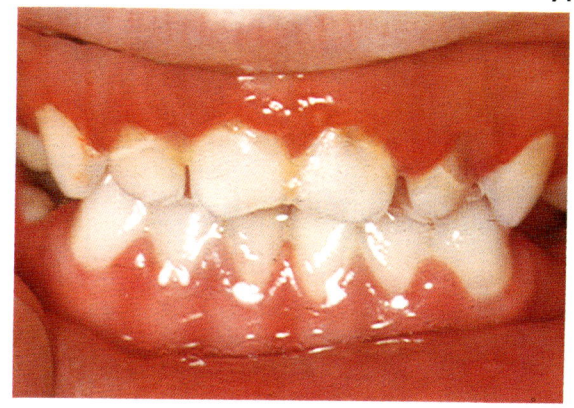

72. The lesions have resolved after ten days. Treatment of the acute phase should, therefore, be symptomatic. Antibiotic therapy may be used to reduce secondary infection. A capsule of tetracycline is broken into about 50cc of water. The resultant suspension is rinsed around the mouth and then swallowed, thus acting both topically and systemically. Tetracycline is contra-indicated in children under the age of ten years as it causes permanent intrinsic staining of the teeth. One episode of herpes simplex infection results in antibody formation and partial immunity. The patient is subsequently liable to develop secondary herpetic lesions but these are confined to the muco-cutaneous junction of the lips.

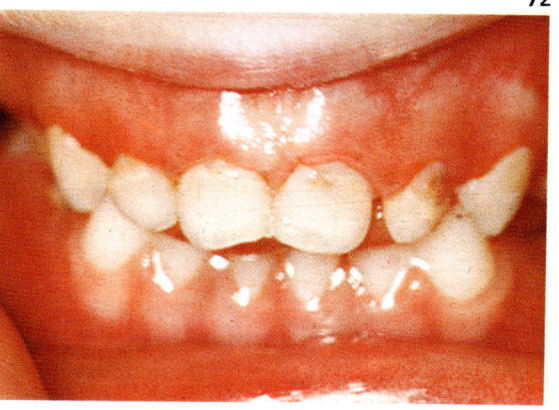

Mucosal lesions

73. Lichen planus is one of the most common dermatological diseases to manifest in the oral cavity. The lesions may occur on the buccal mucosa, tongue, lips, gingivae, floor of the mouth and palate. Four types of lesion are described by Jandinski and Shklar (1976); these are (a) papular keratotic (b) vesiculo bullous (c) erosive (d) atrophic. The different clinical presentations of the lesion complicate diagnosis, which should be confirmed by biopsy if there is any doubt.

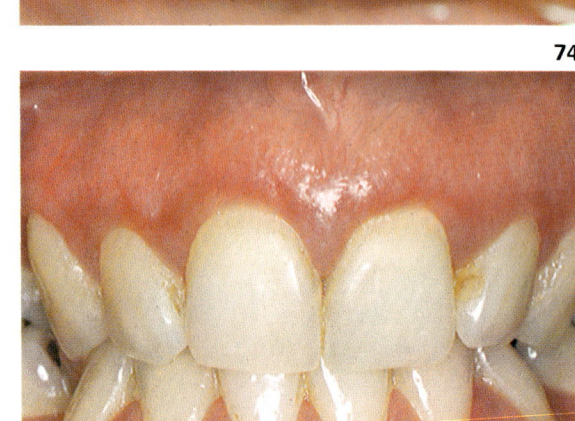

74. Desquamative gingivitis can often be confirmed histologically as atrophic or erosive lichen planus.

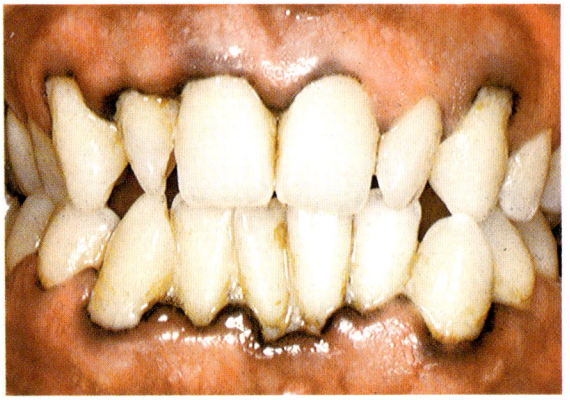

75. Drugs or atmospheric pollutants can also cause gingival pigmentation. This photograph, which was taken several years ago, shows discoloration of the gingiva due to bismuth therapy. The systemic ingestion of other metals or metallic compounds, for example mercury, lead, arsenic or silver, can also cause gingival pigmentation. The discoloration is only found in the presence of marginal inflammation and is probably caused by the precipitation of sulphide salts in the connective tissue. Nowadays industrial pollutants are a more likely cause of gingival pigmentation than drug therapy.

76. After periodontal treatment the discoloration of the gingiva in the above patient has almost disappeared.

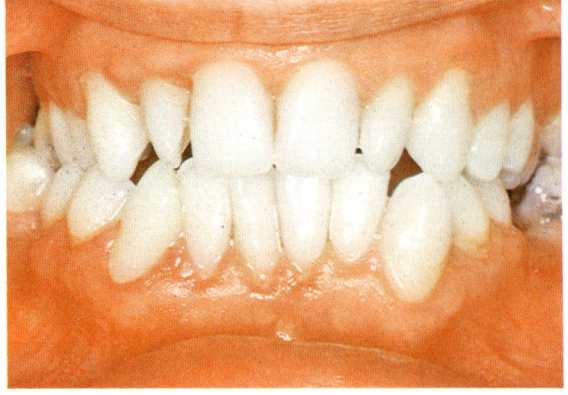

Mucosal lesions

77. Pigmentation of the gingiva is seen most commonly as a racial characteristic (**8**). Local pigmentation, however, can be caused by silver amalgam particles becoming lodged in the tissues during extraction or other oral surgery procedures. In this case the patient had a retrograde root treatment performed some years ago in an unsuccessful attempt to save the right central incisor.

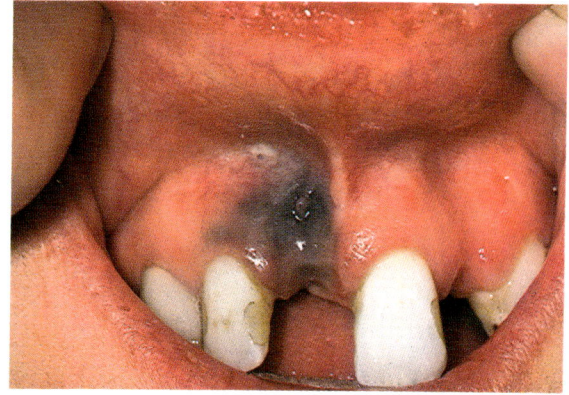

78. The radiograph demonstrates the amalgam particles within the tissues. The area was treated by a gingival graft (**240, 241**).

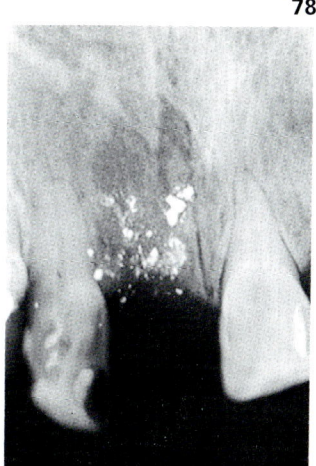

There are many other systemic and dermatological diseases which may give rise to oral lesions. These are covered in texts on oral pathology.

6. Acute periodontal conditions

Acute necrotising ulcerative gingivitis

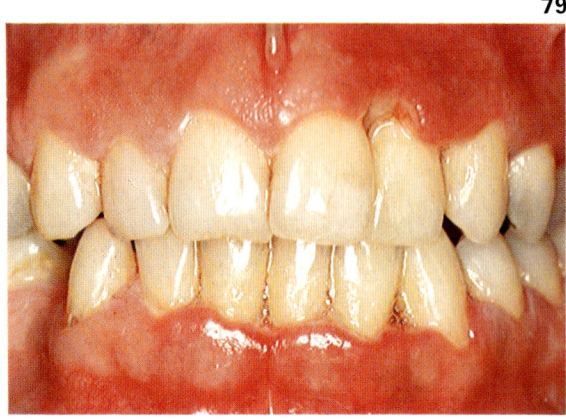

79. Acute necrotising ulcerative gingivitis (ANUG), or Vincent's gingivitis, typically presents in young adults. There is necrosis and ulceration of the interdental papillae and the adjacent gingival margins may also be involved. The symptoms include pain, bleeding from the gingiva, and halitosis. In severe cases there may be pyrexia and submandibular lymphadenopathy. The regions most commonly involved are the lower anterior gingiva, and areas where plaque tends to be retained, for example, the opercula over lower third molars.

80. This is a gram stained smear from a patient with ANUG; there are numerous spirochaetes and fusiform bacteria. The pathology is probably caused by a complex interaction between several species of microorganisms including *Borrelia vincentii* and other spirochaetes, *Fusobacterium nucleatum* and *Bacteroides melaninogenicus*.

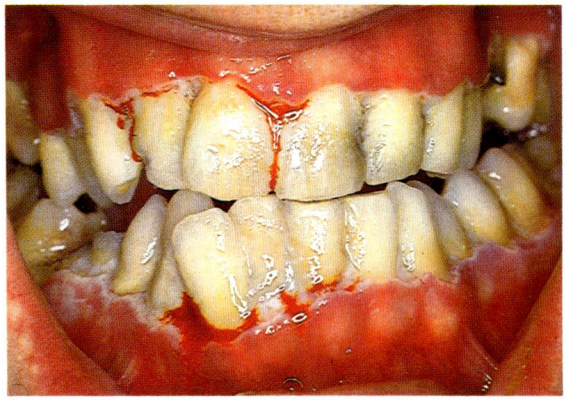

81. Factors predisposing to ANUG include chronic gingivitis, bad oral hygiene, tobacco smoking, and periods of stress. Recurrence is common unless plaque control is instituted.

Acute necrotising ulcerative gingivitis

82. The acute symptoms respond readily to systemic metronidazole or penicillin (Duckworth *et al* 1966). Hydrogen peroxide mouthwash may also be used during the acute phase. Removal of gross deposits should commence immediately. Thorough scaling, and plaque control measures by the patient are brought into operation as soon as the acute symptoms have resolved.

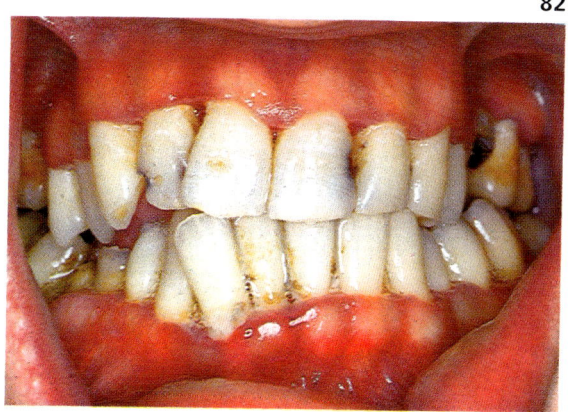

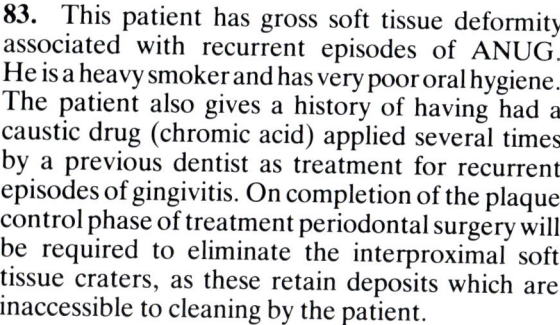

83. This patient has gross soft tissue deformity associated with recurrent episodes of ANUG. He is a heavy smoker and has very poor oral hygiene. The patient also gives a history of having had a caustic drug (chromic acid) applied several times by a previous dentist as treatment for recurrent episodes of gingivitis. On completion of the plaque control phase of treatment periodontal surgery will be required to eliminate the interproximal soft tissue craters, as these retain deposits which are inaccessible to cleaning by the patient.

Acute periodontal abscess

84. A periodontal abscess is caused by a local increase in the concentration of plaque microorganisms within a pocket. On this patient the abscess has perforated the buccal pocket wall and is pointing in the vestibule.

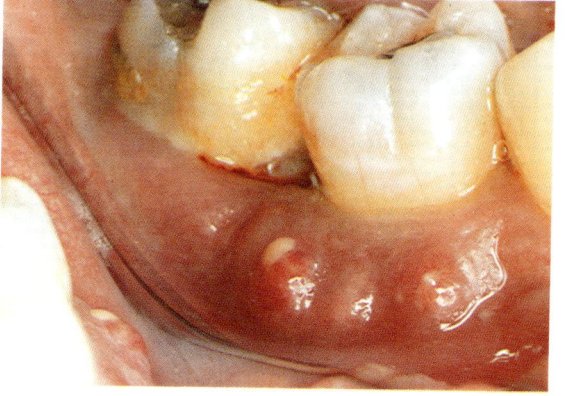

85. The factors predisposing to abscess formation include deep infrabony pockets and, in the case of multirooted teeth, furcation involvement (Miyasato 1975). An additional factor is direct trauma to the soft tissue (**251**).

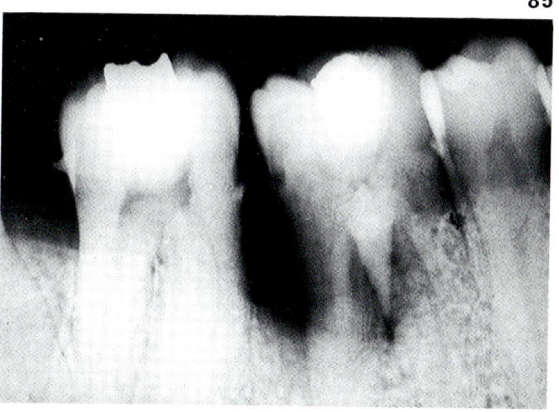

Acute periodontal abscess

86. A periodontal abscess may track through both soft and hard tissues. For example on this patient there is a sinus on the labial aspect of the left upper anterior teeth.

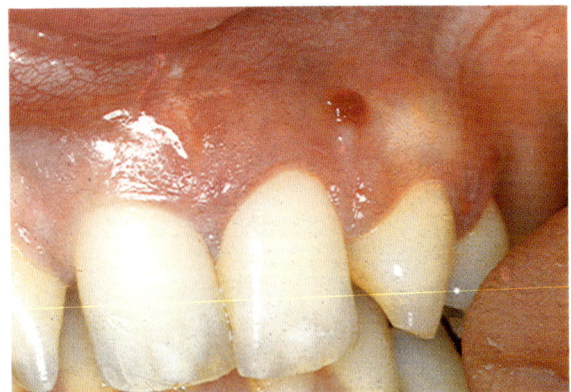

87. The radiograph shows no evidence of a periapical lesion. All the anterior teeth give a positive response to pulp testing. There is rarefaction of bone on the distal aspect of the lateral incisor tooth.

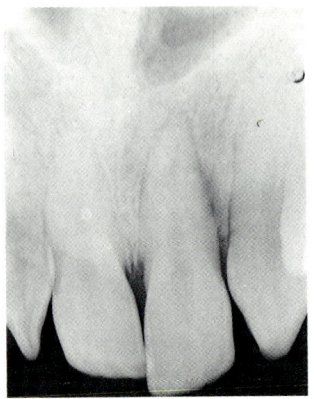

88. On the palatal aspect there is a 6mm pocket, the associated periodontal abscess is tracking between the lateral incisor and the canine. The treatment of the acute symptoms for this patient include incising and opening out of the labial sinus to achieve drainage and curettage of the palatal pocket. The patient is instructed in the use of hot salt mouthwash. If there is pyrexia, lymphadenopathy or other manifestation of systemic involvement antibiotic therapy is indicated (Epstein and Scopp 1977). The causative microorganisms should first be investigated however by taking a specimen from a pocket for culture. An antibiotic sensitivity test should be requested. Initially penicillin or erythromycin should be prescribed with the aim of reducing the acute infection. However, the patient's response must be reviewed and if the symptoms persist then the antibiotic will have to be changed to one active against the particular microorganisms, as indicated by the sensitivity test.

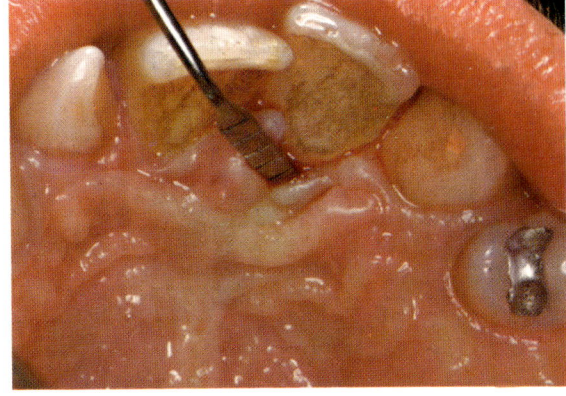

89. Definitive pocket elimination should be performed soon after the resolution of the acute phase or there is the danger of recurrence. The inverse bevel flap procedure is being used to gain access (Chapter 12). The infra-bony defect on the palatal aspect is curetted to remove the chronic inflammatory tissue. This bone defect is to be treated by osteoplasty and regeneration techniques (Chapter 13).

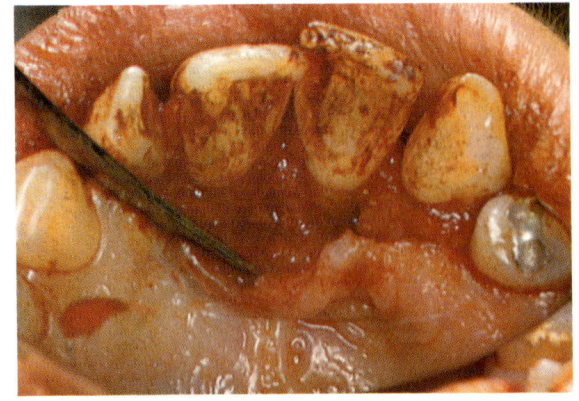

Acute periodontal abscess

90. The symptoms have resolved and the pockets have been eliminated by the use of this treatment regime. The porcelain jacket crowns on the lateral incisors were placed subsequently to improve aesthetics.

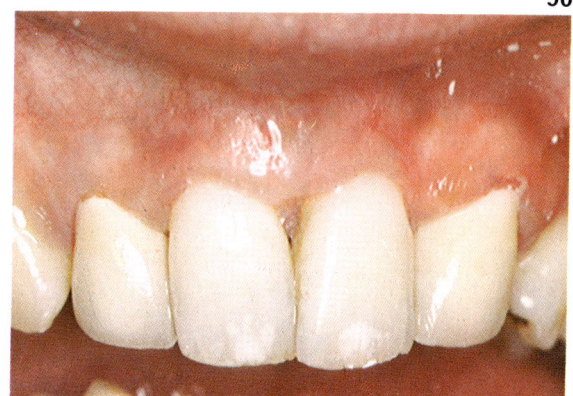

91. This patient has a generalised acute inflammation involving the gingival tissues. There is discharge from many of the pockets. An acute exacerbation of pre-existing periodontal disease as seen here may be due to a change in the concentration or virulence of the microorganisms, or to a reduction in host resistance as for example with acute leukaemia. The latter must be excluded by haematological tests.

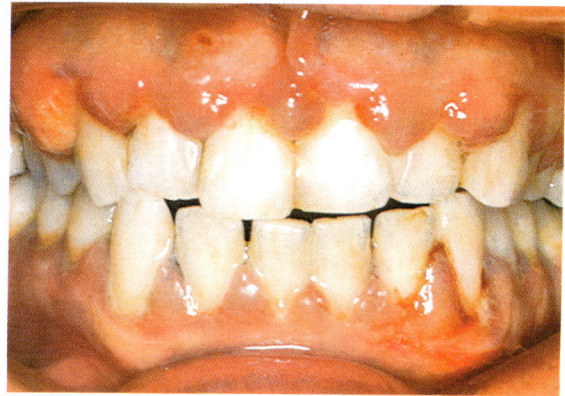

Acute periapical abscess

92. The acute periapical abscess usually points on the alveolar mucosa. Less commonly it may track subperiosteally or via the periodontal ligament; it then may achieve drainage into the gingival sulcus or point on the gingiva. It is differentiated from a periodontal abscess by vitality tests and by radiographic assessment.

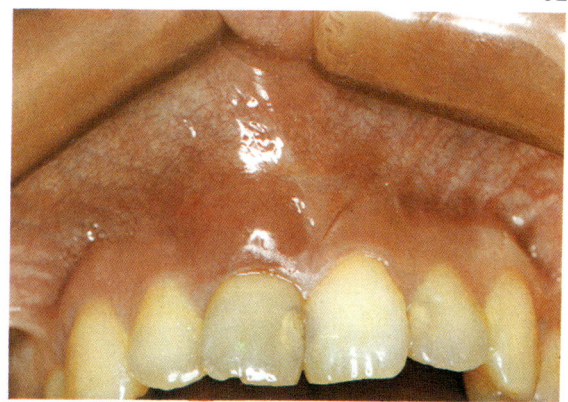

93. The radiograph of this tooth shows a periapical radiolucency. There is a deep silicate restoration which probably caused the original pulp injury. Access into the pulp chamber for drainage has been achieved via the palatal aspect of the tooth.

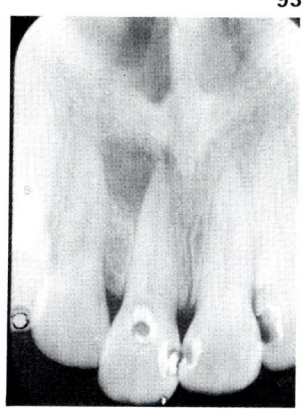

7. The assessment of the periodontal patient (see Appendix 3)

The history

A thorough case history provides the relevant background to the present dental condition of the patient, enabling the clinical picture to be related to any predisposing factors and to previous treatment. The taking of a history is therefore fundamental to accurate diagnosis.

Presenting complaint
The patient is first questioned as to whether he has any symptoms from his gums or teeth. The patient with periodontal disease usually has few complaints as pain is not a symptom of chronic inflammation. He should be questioned specifically as to whether he has pain, swelling, redness, bleeding, discharge or recession affecting the gums, and whether he has noticed any teeth becoming mobile or teeth drifting out of alignment in the arch.

History of complaint
Further information is sought about the date of onset of symptoms and about subsequent developments, including any previous treatment provided for the condition.

Oral history
The patient is questioned about his past dental treatment. Details concerning previous restorative, prosthetic, orthodontic, periodontic and preventive therapy are obtained. Habits such as tobacco smoking or betel nut chewing which might affect the oral condition are also recorded. A comprehensive diagnosis must be based on a thorough knowledge of the previous oral history.

Oral hygiene methods
Information should be obtained about the frequency and method of toothbrushing and the type of brush used. Similar questions are asked about interproximal cleaning.

Medical history
A detailed medical history is essential. It enables a treatment plan to be developed which is compatible with both the medical background and any drug therapy.

There are also a number of medical conditions which influence the response of the tissues to plaque and are therefore of relevance to the periodontal assessment (Chapter 4). Haematological tests, biopsy or other special tests may be indicated by the patient's history. The patient should be questioned about his present state of health and whether he has had any serious disease. He should be questioned in particular as to whether he has had rheumatic fever, cardiac disease, diabetes or hepatitis; a history of hepatitis will necessitate a blood test for Australia Antigen (Sims 1976). Recent or current drug therapy should be ascertained, together with details of previous treatment in hospital. A history of prolonged bleeding after a surgical procedure or any drug allergy should be noted.

The examination

An extra-oral examination is carried out. The previous case history may direct attention to a particular zone, for example to the temporo-mandibular joints, or to the lymph nodes draining a region. The position of the lips at rest is also assessed (**39** and **249**).

The intra-oral tissues are now examined. A complete oral examination of all patients is important so that if a malignant lesion is present it may be diagnosed and treated early. It is also important to recognise other mucosal lesions as the same pathological condition may be manifested in the gingiva, for example lichen planus may be present on both the mucosa and gingiva (**73** and **74**). All the mucosal surfaces in the mouth are examined, including the pharynx, fauces, soft and hard palate, tongue, floor of the mouth, vestibule and buccal mucosa.

The attached gingiva, the marginal gingivae and the papillae are assessed. A note is made of change in colour, shape, consistency or contour. The presence of a frenum which encroaches onto the attached gingiva is noted (**14**). Where there is enhanced gingival response to plaque deposits special tests are indicated to ascertain whether there is a systemic cause for this manifestation. These tests may include haemoglobin concentration, differential white blood cell count, blood film for abnormal cells, blood glucose concentration, etc (**49** and **51**).

The examination

94. The periodontal pockets are measured on all the surfaces of the teeth with a graduated probe and are recorded in the patient's notes. Either a full periodontal chart can be completed as illustrated, or for the less complicated case a more basic chart can be used (Appendix 3).

The chart is completed as follows: teeth which have been extracted are shaded in. Restorations and cavities are marked on the occlusal views on the chart, and overhanging margins of restorations can be indicated on the lateral views. Any teeth which have had endodontic treatment are noted and a record is made of crowned teeth, pontics or removable prostheses.

The soft tissues are then assessed. The periodontal probe is used to measure the position of the gingival margin in relation to the enamel-cement junction at the mesial, mid-marginal and distal of each tooth. The points are marked on the chart; each of the grid lines represent two millimetres. A blue line representing the gingival margin, is used to join these points.

The clinical depths of the pockets are measured from the gingival margin at each of the above three points. Where the depths exceed two millimetres they are marked on the chart by a vertical red line.

The position of the muco-gingival junction in relation to the gingival margin is measured and marked in with a broken line. This enables the position of the base of the pockets to be related to the muco-gingival junction. Frenal and high muscle attachments are outlined on the chart. Asterisks are used to indicate furcation involvements.

The final procedure is to indicate irregularities in tooth position by arrows, for example over-eruption drifting or rotation of teeth. Open contacts are represented by parallel lines.

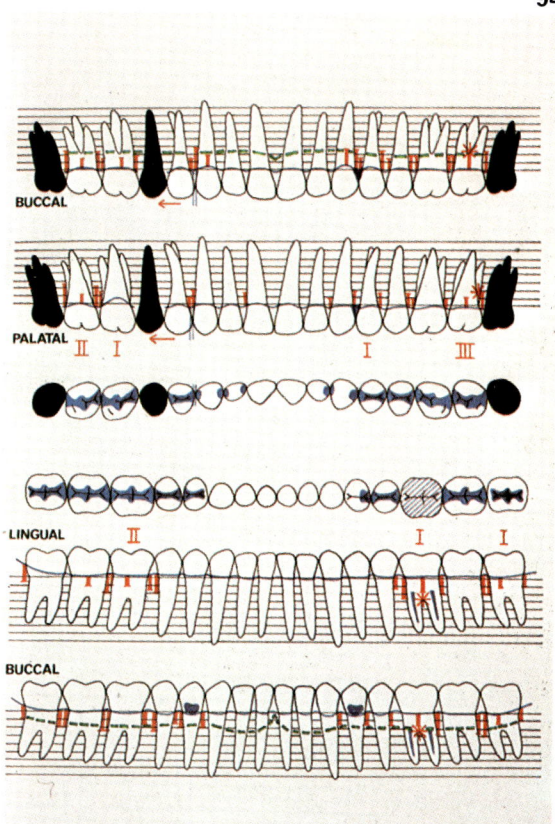

The examination

95. Mobility is assessed by applying a bucco-lingual force to the tooth with two instruments. It is scored:
- 0 Physiological mobility
- I Less than 1mm movement
- II 1mm movement
- III Over 1mm movement with vertical movement in socket.

Tooth deposits

The presence and distribution of plaque and supragingival and subgingival calculus is noted. One of the indices may be used to obtain a precise record, but this is not obligatory for treatment purposes (Appendix 2).

Occlusion

The Angle's classification is recorded. The occlusion is assessed with the mandible in the retruded contact position (**273**), in the intercuspal position, in lateral excursion and in protrusion. The articulation between these positions is checked and interferences noted. The degree of mobility is correlated with these findings. The patient is questioned about bruxism, clenching or other habits likely to exert excessive forces on the periodontium

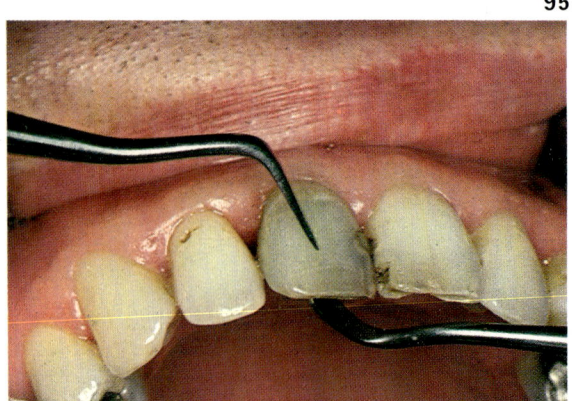

Radiographic assessment

96. Bite wing radiographs provide a good view of interproximal bone provided bone loss is not advanced. However, additional views are required of the periapical region.

The information obtained from the case history and examination is used to compile a treatment plan. This should be designed so that the various aspects of treatment are coordinated (see Appendix 4).

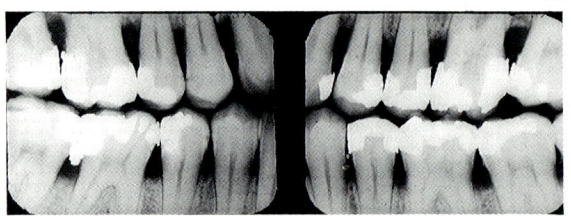

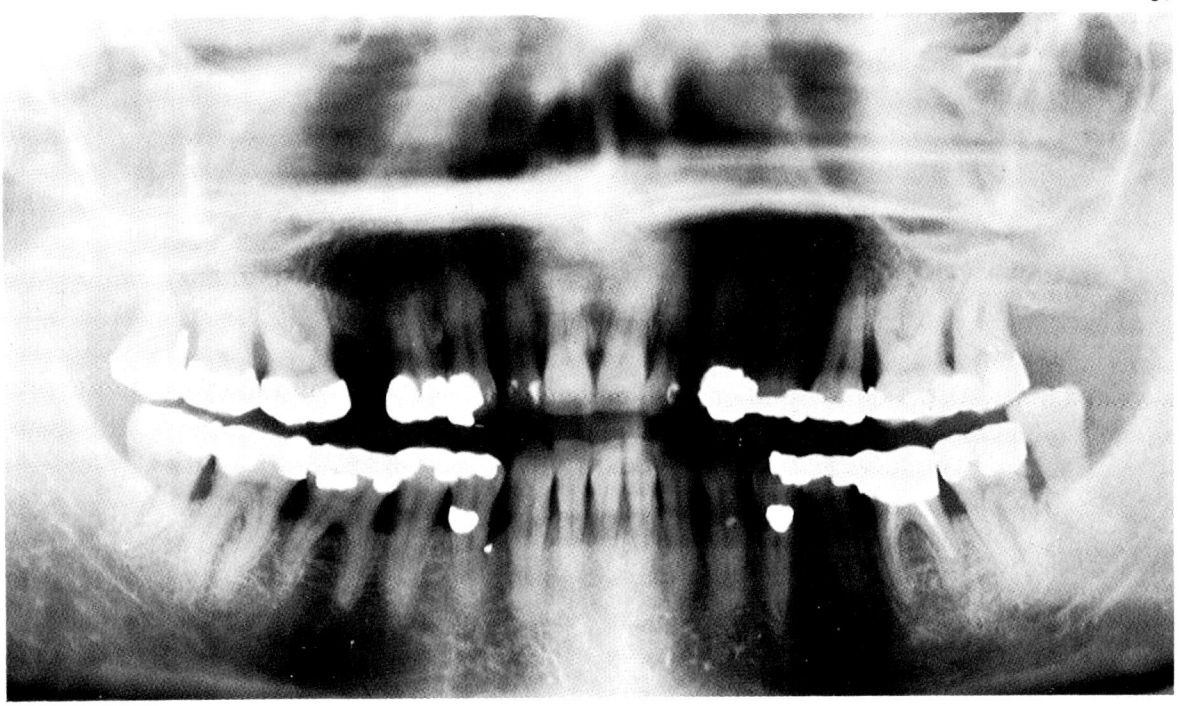

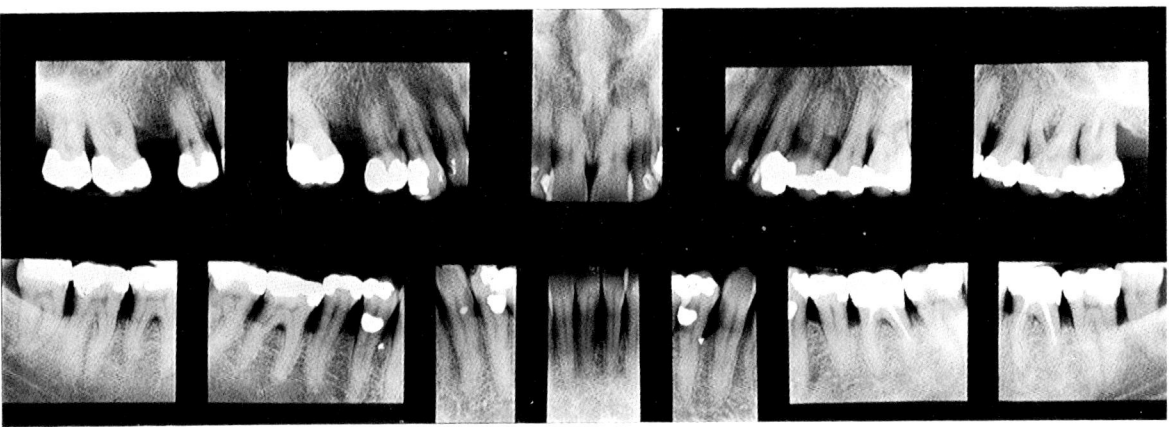

97. Panoramic radiographs provide a general view of the oral structures. They give an indication of the amount of bone destruction, but they are not suitable for accurate assessment of the degree of bone loss associated with individual teeth, as there is severe distortion and the outline of the bone margin is often not clear due to superimposition of intervening structures.

98. A variety of radiographic techniques may be used for detailed periodontal assessment. Periapical radiographs taken by long cone paralleling technique, as shown here, are preferred as these show the least distortion. For clarity only a restricted number of films are illustrated; a full mouth series comprises 14 films. Where facilities are not available for the paralleling technique conventional periapical views are acceptable. These radiographs are from the same patient as illustrated in **94** and **97**. The upper right third molar tooth was extracted after the orthopantomograph had been taken, as it was causing pain due to a periodontal abscess.

8. *The control of dental plaque*

Introduction

The control of dental plaque is the basis of both the prevention and treatment of periodontal disease (Suomi *et al* 1969, Strahan *et al* 1977). The objective is to establish a routine of oral hygiene which is of a sufficiently high standard to result in the achievement and maintenance of a healthy mouth.

Motivation

The first phase of the plaque control programme is the reinforcement of motivation. Patients respond to various goals and an appropriate theme must be selected for each individual. It should be emphasised to the patient that the prevention of periodontal disease maintains the good appearance of the mouth, preserves good masticatory function, and reduces the need for periodontal and restorative treatment in the future.

Education

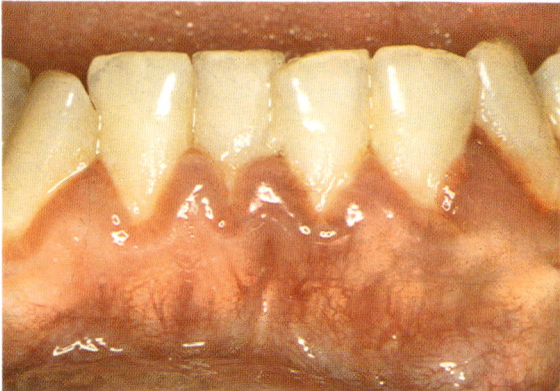

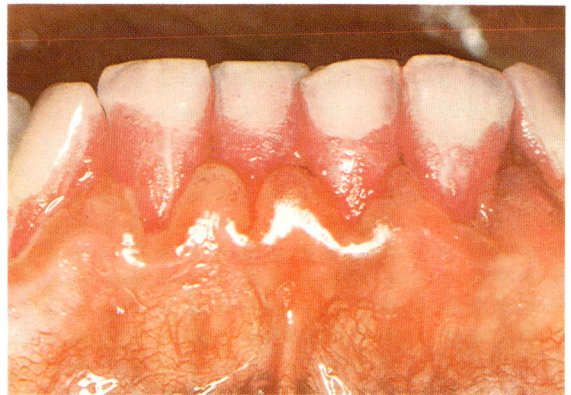

99. This girl is 22 years old and has early periodontitis associated with generalised plaque deposits. She is informed in simple terms about plaque and the damage it causes to the teeth and the supporting structures. The signs of periodontal disease are demonstrated in her own mouth, so that she can see and be encouraged by the subsequent improvement in the periodontal condition.

100. A disclosing agent is used to stain the deposits and she is then shown that the presence of plaque is associated with gingival inflammation and pocketing.

Instruction

Clear information must be given about which type of toothbrush and which interproximal cleaning aid are to be used. Samples of these should be provided to prevent any misunderstanding. Disclosing tablets and a mouth mirror may also be supplied so that plaque deposits may be seen even in the less accessible areas of the mouth. The present patient has been instructed to clean her teeth at least twice a day – after breakfast and before going to bed, at night.

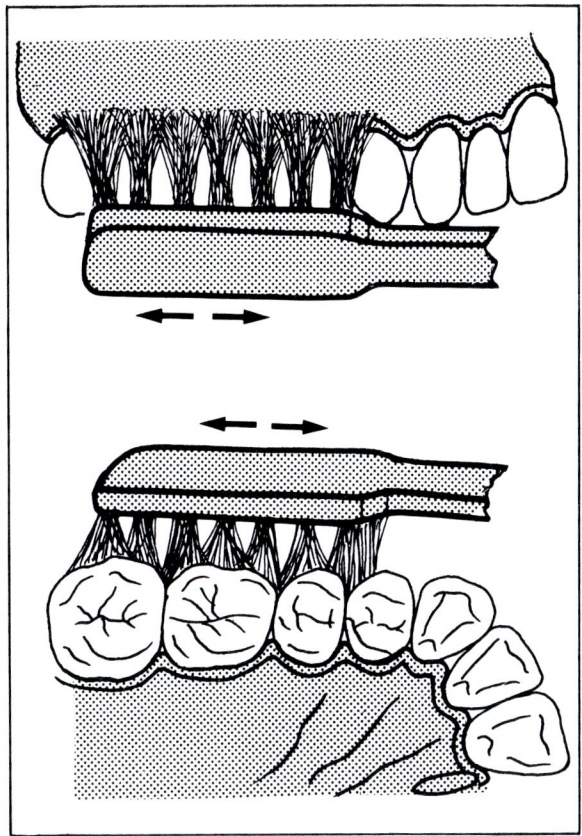

101. The Bass toothbrushing technique has proved to be a versatile procedure for removing plaque even when the arch form or the gingival contour is not ideal. For the Bass technique the brush head is positioned over the dento-gingival junction with the filaments angled into the sulcus at 45° to the long axes of the teeth. The brush is activated with a mesio-distal vibratory movement.

The electric toothbrush is useful for handicapped patients or for patients with poor manual dexterity. Some patients prefer the electric toothbrush to the manual one and the two techniques appear to be equally effective (Bergenholtz 1972). The patient must be instructed to apply the filaments of the brush to the gingival margins and to follow a set sequence when using the electric brush.

102. The oral hygiene procedures should first be demonstrated on models. A systematic procedure for brushing must be established, each quadrant being cleaned in three segments on the labial and three segments on the lingual. Following this the occlusal surfaces are brushed.

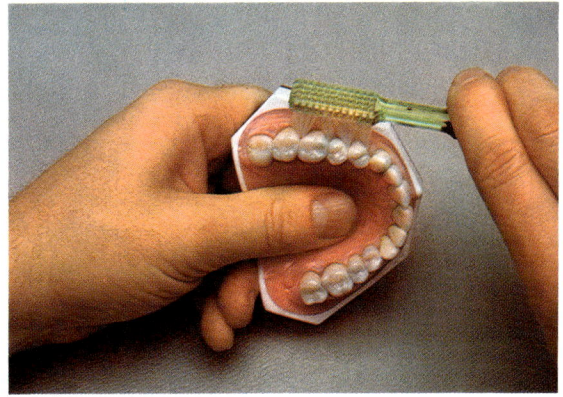

103. The procedures are now carried out in the patient's own mouth, so that she can see that the disclosed plaque is being removed. The operator is demonstrating toothbrushing on one side of the mouth.

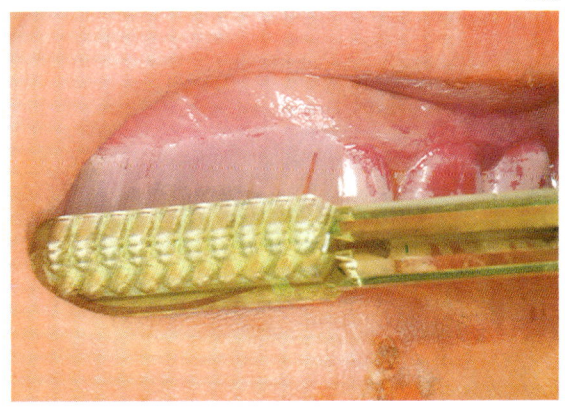

Instruction

104. The patient then attempts to repeat the procedure on the other side. The instructor should take the patient's hand and guide it in the correct movements. The patient can in this way recognise the correct positions of the brush filaments on the gingiva by tactile sensation.

Interproximal cleaning may be carried out with either floss or triangular wood sticks. Floss has the advantage that it cleans all the interproximal surfaces including the contact points. Wood sticks are quicker and require less manual dexterity, however they should only be used when recession of the interproximal papillae has resulted in there being sufficient space for them to be used without causing trauma (Bergenholtz *et al* 1974).

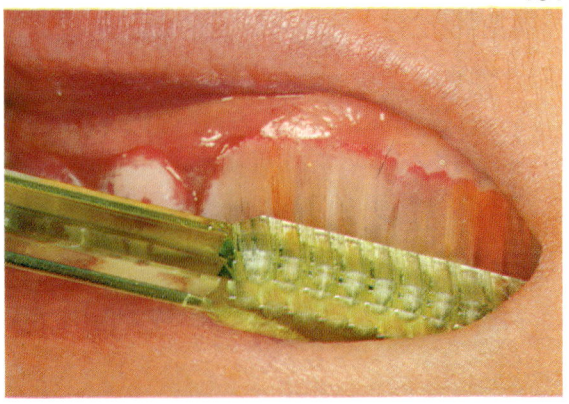

105. Interproximal cleaning is now demonstrated in the mouth. The ends of the floss are wound around the middle finger of each hand, leaving the thumb and forefinger free to guide the working section. The floss is passed through the contact point with a bucco-lingual sliding action.

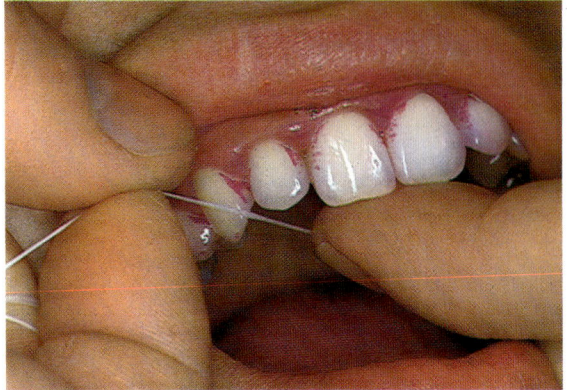

106. The distal surface is cleaned by bringing the floss to the base of the sulcus and wrapping the floss around the tooth.

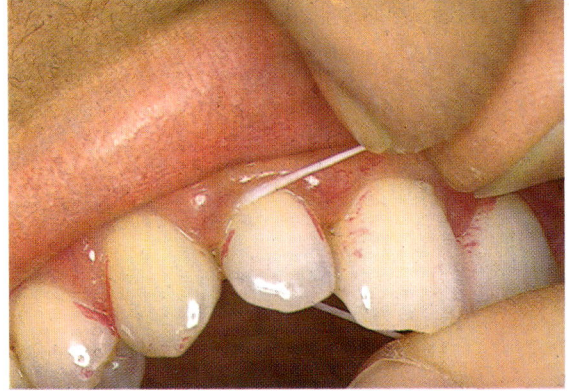

107. The floss is withdrawn using a vertical wiping action. This is repeated until the surface is free of stained plaque.

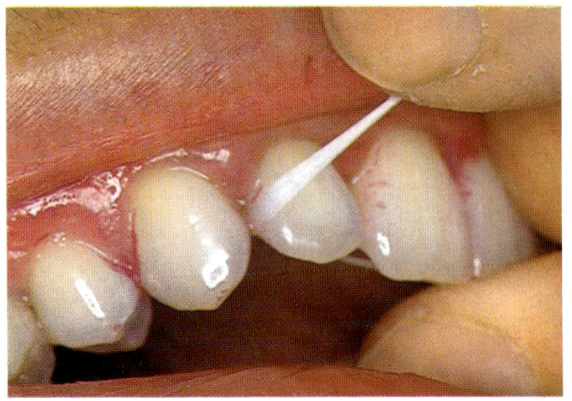

Instruction

108. The floss is then brought across the embrasure to clean the mesial tooth surface. Each interspace is then cleaned in the same way in a systematic order.

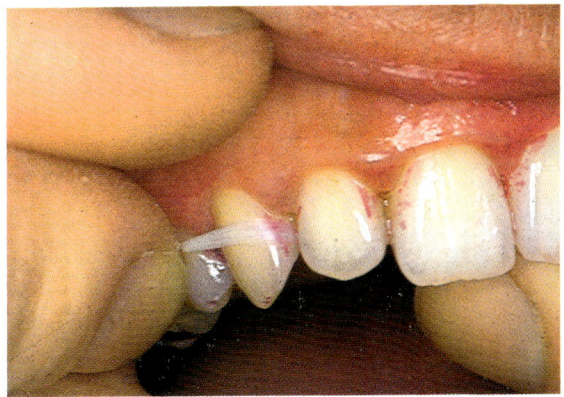

109. Where difficulty is experienced in reaching the back of the mouth a floss holder may be used.

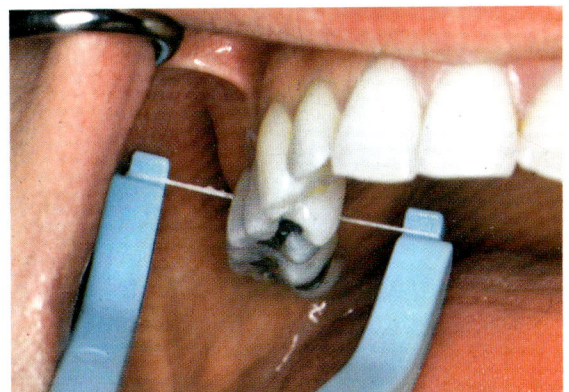

110. Floss threaders should be used for cleaning the pontics and retainers of bridgework.

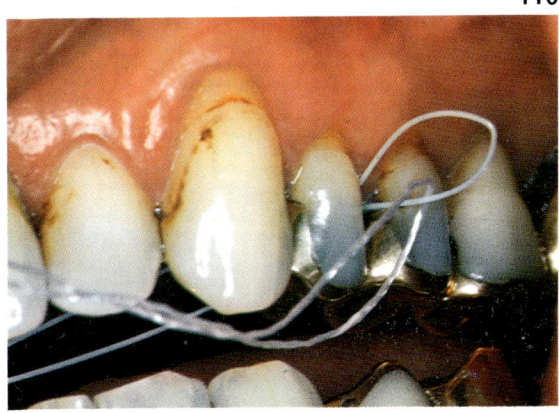

111. Interdental wood sticks are an alternative to floss. A variety of sizes are available and an appropriate one should be selected for the size of the interproximal spaces. The wood sticks are used with a bucco-lingual rubbing action against the interdental tooth surfaces and papillae. The angulation of the wood stick is important and this must be adjusted so that the gingivae on the lingual aspect are not traumatised.

Following oral hygiene instruction all the teeth are scaled and polished, and the margins of restorations which are in contact with the gingiva are smoothed. The completion of scaling may take several visits (Chapter 9).

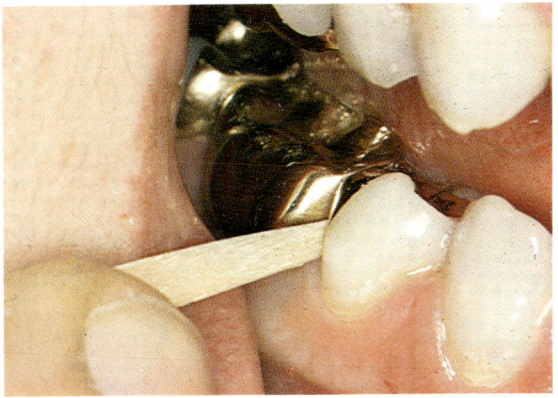

Reinforcement of plaque control

112. Progress is reassessed at each visit. At this stage we are seeing the same patient four weeks after the commencement of treatment (compare with **99** and **100**). She is shown the improvement in the periodontal condition and given encouragement.

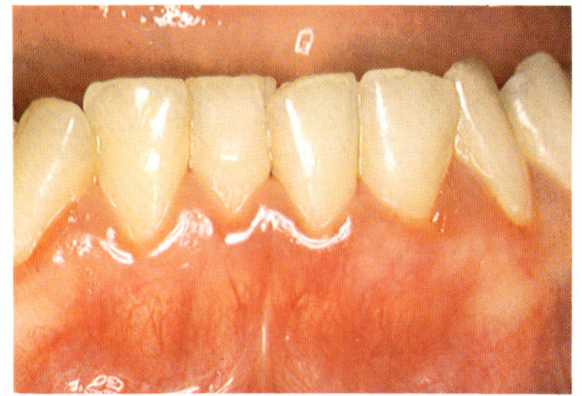

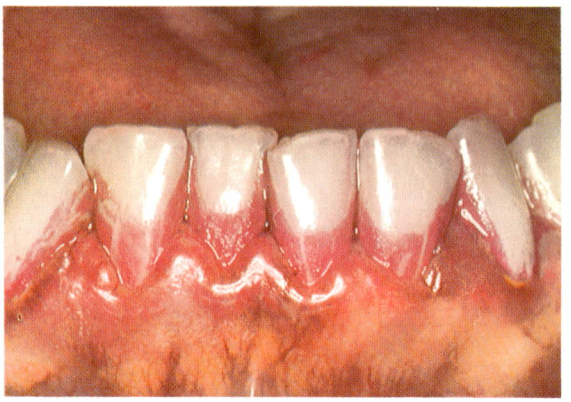

113. Plaque deposits are disclosed again and the areas requiring particular attention emphasised. Further demonstration of the oral hygiene procedures is given, and the patient's own performance observed and any necessary correction given.

114. Over a four month period there has been resolution of inflammation as a result of the excellent plaque control maintained by the patient. She must be informed about the need to maintain this high standard of oral hygiene. At recall visits the co-operation must be assessed and the instruction again reinforced.

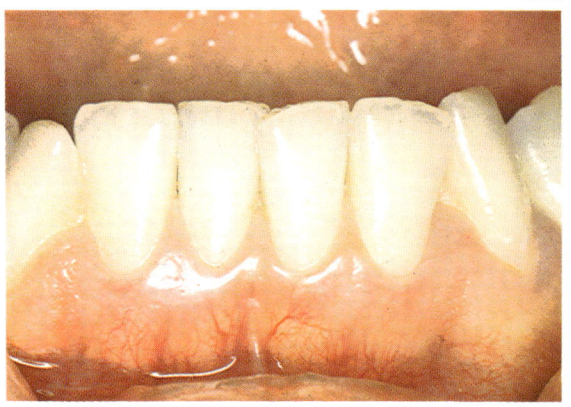

Supplementary aids

115. In general the technique of plaque control should be kept as simple as possible, however there are situations where additional procedures may help. There are a variety of interproximal brushes which are of value if there are wide interproximal spaces and difficult tissue contours to clean. They should be demonstrated in the patient's own mouth.

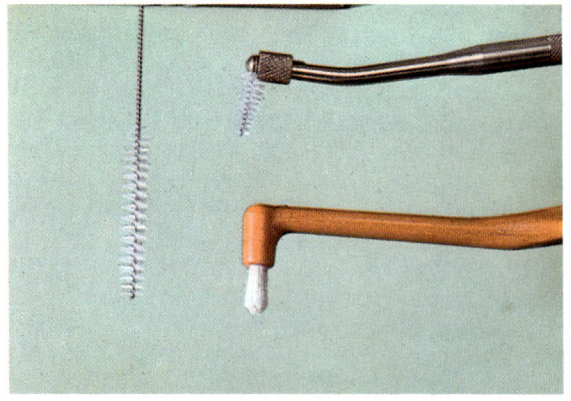

Supplementary aids

116. Pulsed water jet instruments are available from several manufacturers. It has been found that the regular use of water lavage brings about a reduction in gingival inflammation by diluting the concentration of plaque metabolites; modified bacterial cells however still remain adhering to the tooth surface (Brady *et al* 1973). Water jet instruments may be used for cleaning fixed orthodontic appliances and temporary splints, and they are of value to handicapped patients with poor manual dexterity.

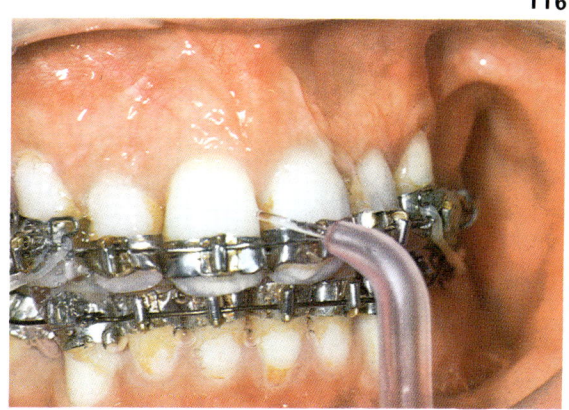

117. Löe and Rindom Schiøtt (1970) have shown that a 0.2 per cent solution of chlorhexidine used as a mouthwash is effective at preventing plaque growth on clean tooth surfaces in the absence of pocketing. Chlorhexidine is useful for controlling plaque formation when the gingivae are painful, for example where there is acute inflammation and after surgery.

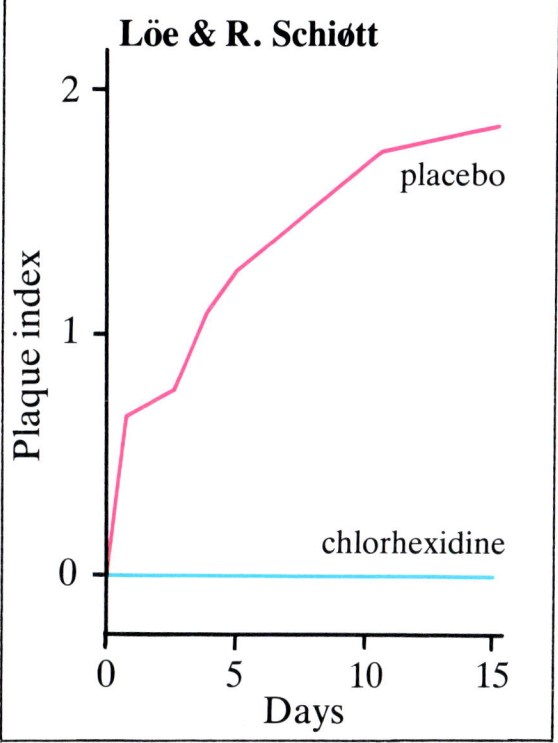

118. The main problem with the use of chlorhexidine is that a brown stain tends to form on the teeth. The solution has a bitter taste, and some patients complain of a 'burning' sensation from the mucosa after a period of using the mouthwash.

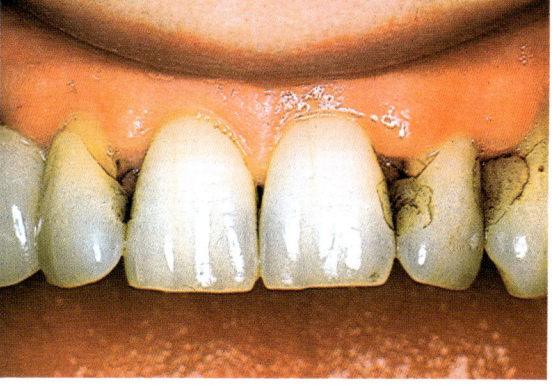

9. Scaling and polishing

The objectives of scaling and polishing are to remove soft deposits and calculus, and to smooth and polish the tooth surfaces and the margins of restorations where these are related to the gingiva. These procedures aid subsequent plaque removal by the patient. Where there are extensive deposits of subgingival calculus, scaling may have to be carried out over several visits. Local analgesia may be used where necessary. In the previous chapter a patient was presented for whom a plaque control programme and treatment by scaling and polishing resulted in resolution of inflammation. The technique and instrumentation for the scaling and polishing procedure are to be described in this chapter.

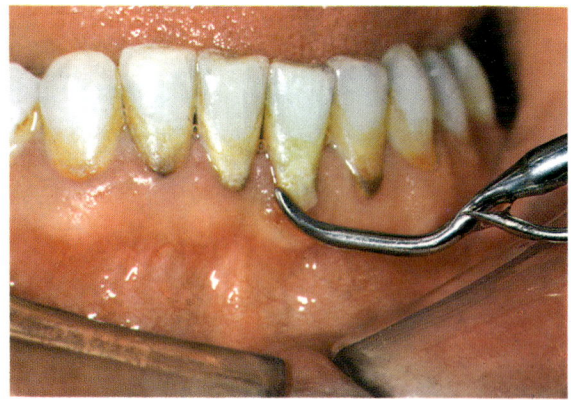

119. Gross deposits may be removed either with ultrasonic scalers (Suppipat 1974) or with hand instruments. Many patients prefer the high frequency vibrations and lighter forces associated with the use of ultrasonic instrumentation. The water spray not only cools the tip but also removes debris. However, some patients find that the cold water spray causes pain where there is exposed dentine; and others dislike the sensation produced by the oscillating tip.

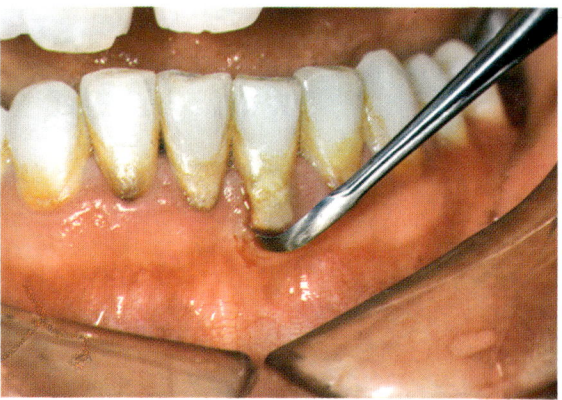

120. Alternatively a relatively robust hand instrument, for example a Cumine scaler, may be used for removing the gross supragingival deposits. However, manual scaling takes longer and is more tiring for the operator.

121. The removal of residual deposits is undertaken with hand instruments as these provide better tactile sensation. The sickle scaler may be used for moderate amounts of supragingival and for relatively superficial subgingival deposits.

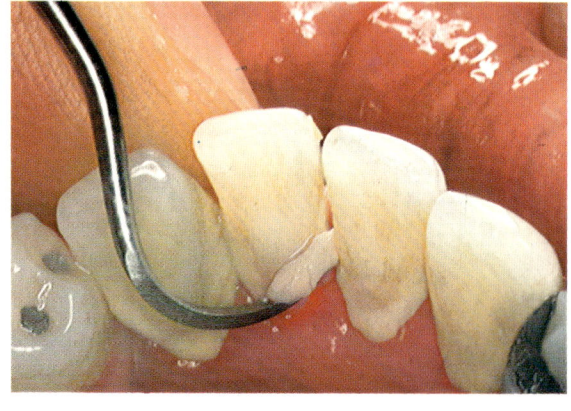

Scaling and polishing

122. The blade of the instrument is triangular in shape, with the result that the non-working edge of the blade tends to traumatise the crevicular epithelium if an attempt is made to remove deeper subgingival calculus.

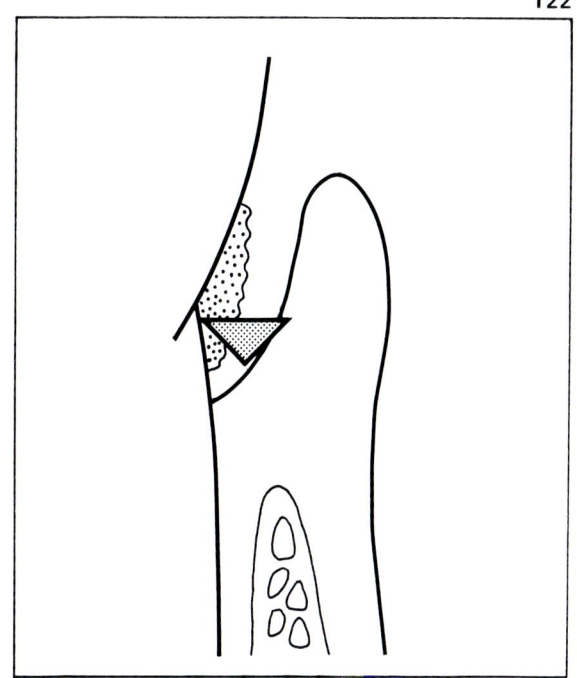

123. Subgingival calculus is difficult to detect. The presence of deposits may be suspected where there is persistent localised inflammation in spite of good oral hygiene. Relatively superficial calculus may sometimes be seen by displacing the gingival wall of the pocket with an air jet or with a periodontal probe. Interproximal deposits can often be seen on radiographs. The fundamental technique for the detection of subgingival calculus however is by probing. A Cross calculus probe, as illustrated, may be used for this. Calculus is recognised by the presence of an upper edge, a relatively rough surface and a lower edge. In contrast a defective margin usually only has one edge, and a carious cavity is felt as an indentation in the tooth.

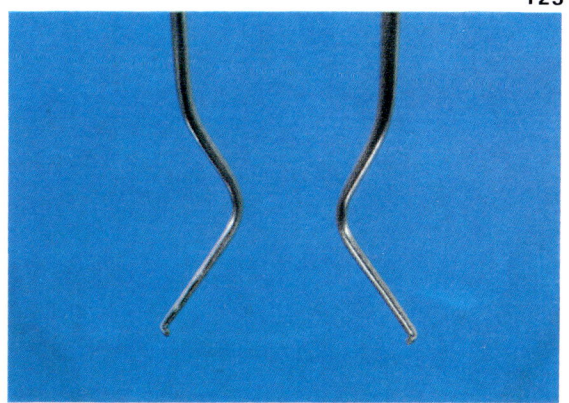

124. Periodontal hoes are used for the removal of tenacious calculus deposits. There are four hoes in each set, to provide the correct angulation for each tooth surface. The instruments are used with vertical overlapping strokes.

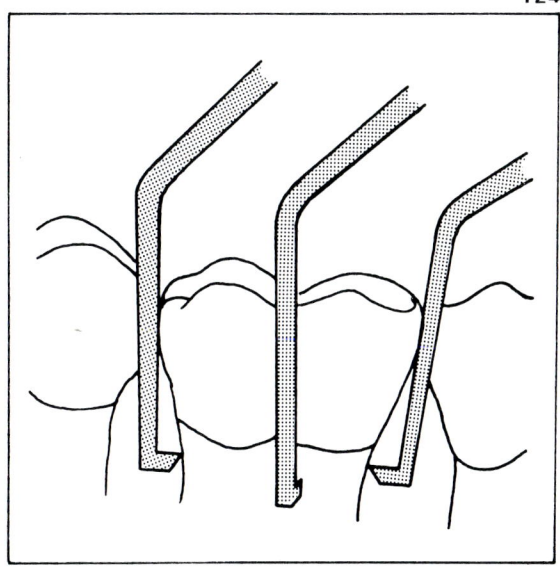

Scaling and polishing

125. The hoe is passed gently into the pocket until the upper edge of the calculus is felt. The blade is then moved horizontally away from the root surface and pushed gently in an apical direction over the surface of the calculus, which is rough to instrumentation. The blade can be felt to engage under the apical edge of the calculus near the base of the pocket. Pressure is applied against the root surface as the instrument is withdrawn, the deposits being removed by this planing action.

The design of the tip of the hoe prevents the removal of deep deposits when these are closely related to the base of the pocket. Considerable pressure is exerted at the cutting edge over a small area of tooth. This tends to cause a gouged surface, and a broader bladed instrument such as a curette should be used after the hoe to smooth the surface.

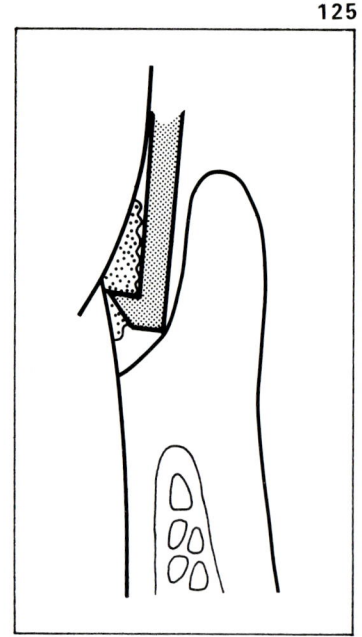

126. Curettes may be used for the removal of both supra and subgingival deposits, and for smoothing the tooth surface. Their use on the soft tissues is described in Chapter 10. Several designs are available; the Gracey and Goldman-Fox instruments are illustrated.

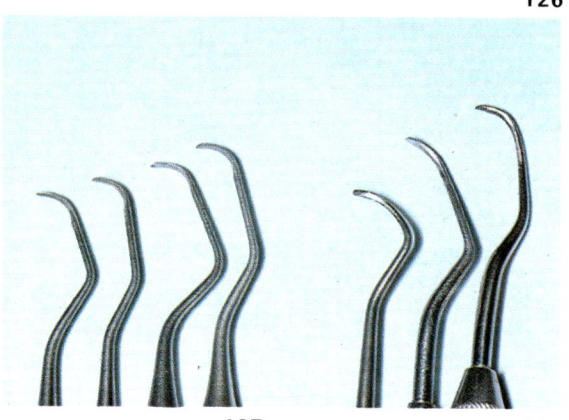

127. The curette is inserted into the pocket with the flat surface of the blade parallel to the root surface. The presence of calculus is confirmed when the instrument abuts against the upper edge of the deposit and by the relative roughness of its surface.

128. When the curette engages below the lower edge of the calculus the angulation of the instrument is changed so that the cutting edge is brought into action. Pressure is applied to the blade as it is withdrawn.

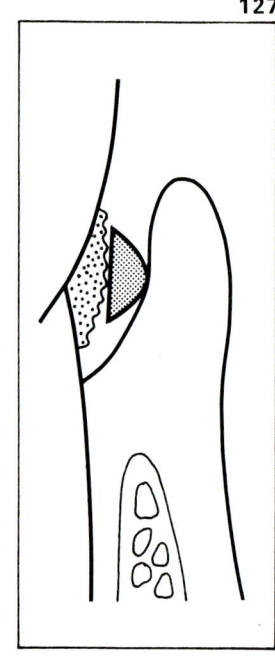
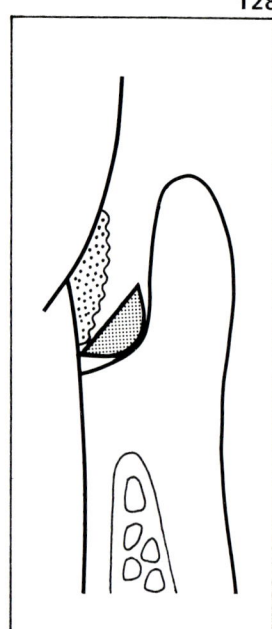

Scaling and polishing

129. The chisel scaler is designed for the removal of supra and subgingival deposits in the interproximal regions, using a horizontal action. It has a very narrow blade enabling it to be used near the base of the pocket. The instrument must not be applied too far apically or the junctional epithelium may be disrupted.

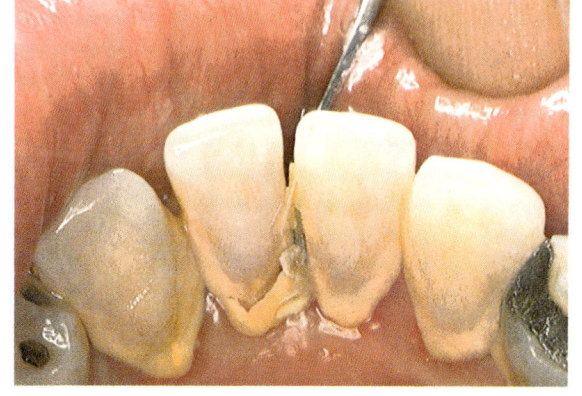

130. The teeth are now polished. A small cup-shaped brush and abrasive paste are used to remove supragingival stains and plaque. A rubber cup with polishing paste is used to remove any roughness and can be used to polish the tooth surfaces within the sulcus.

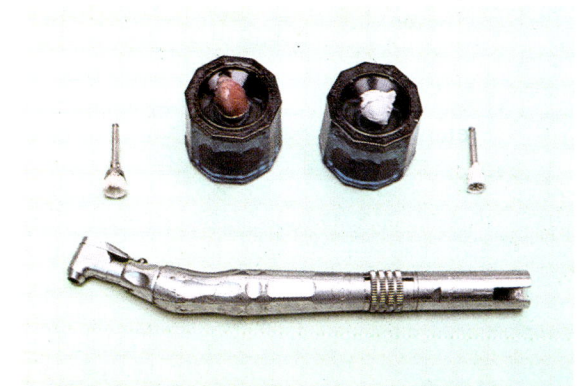

131. The interproximal surfaces are smoothed and polished with fine abrasive strips. The ends should be cut to a point to enable the strips to be passed through the interproximal spaces.

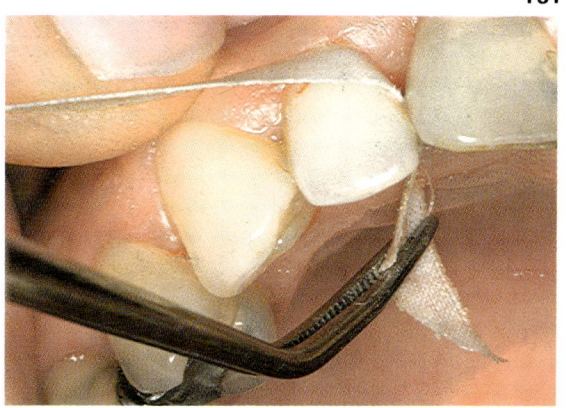

132. Alternatively, a triangular wood stick in a porte-polisher or a reciprocating handpiece with special polishing inserts may be used. This handpiece also has diamond tips which are of value for reducing the overhanging interproximal margins of restorations.

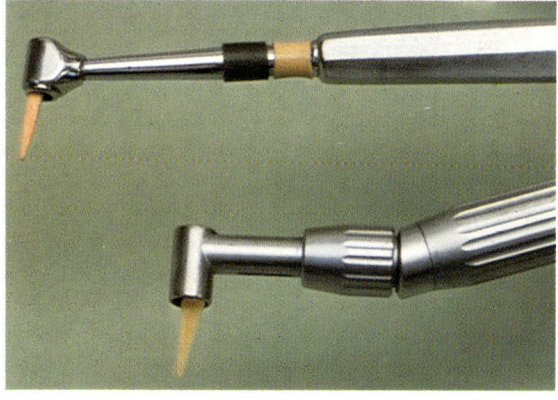

Displacement dressings

133. Where there is severe inflammation and ulceration of the lining of the pocket it may be found that scaling procedures cause profuse bleeding which interferes with the removal of the deposits. This patient has had a crown with imperfect margins on the right central incisor for several years; there is localised proliferation and inflammation confined mainly to this tooth.

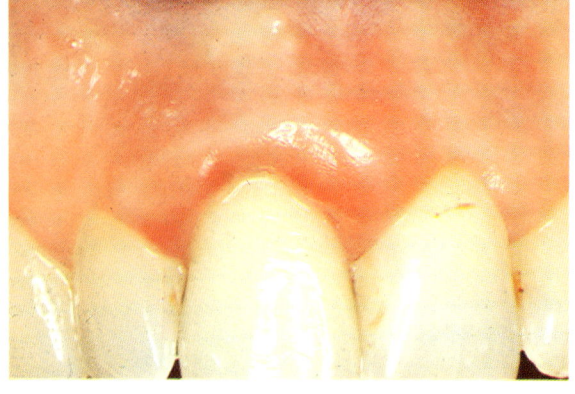

134. The tissues are being displaced with a zinc oxide and eugenol dressing which has been mixed with cotton wool fibres. If necessary this type of dressing may be secured with a floss ligature to increase retention.

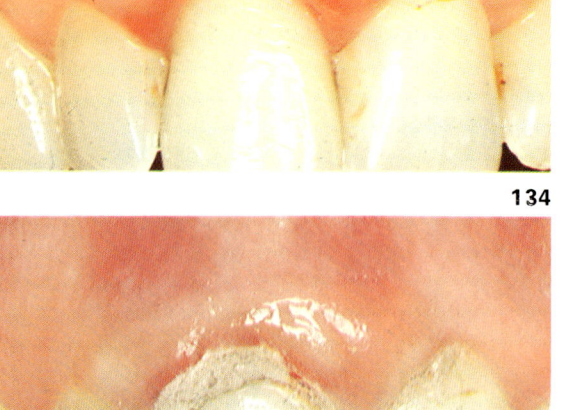

135. After two to three days the dressing is removed. The displacement of the soft tissues has provided access for the removal of deposits and for the contouring of the crown margins.

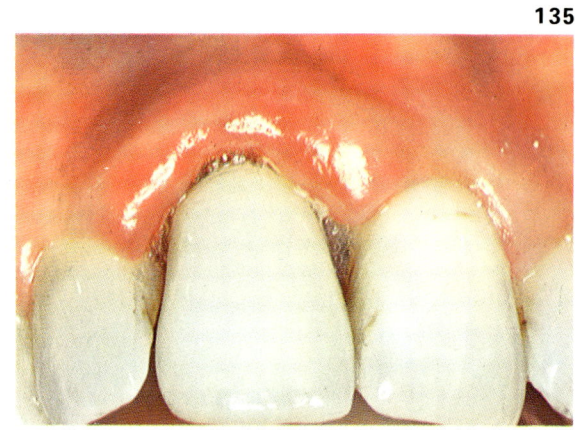

136. One month later there has been considerable reduction in inflammation. Re-examination will be undertaken at subsequent visits to assess the need for further treatment.

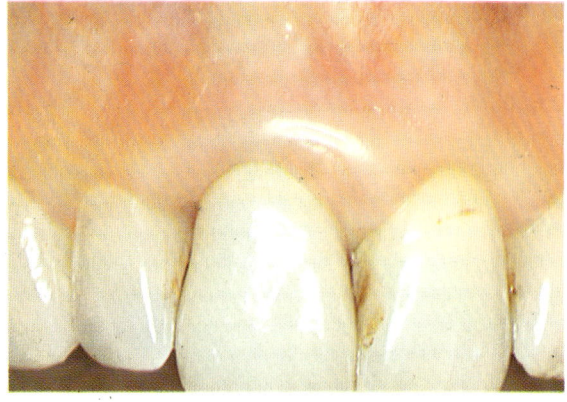

10. Subgingival curettage

Introduction: rationale for surgical treatment

It has been emphasised in Chapters 8 and 9 that plaque control and scaling procedures frequently result in the resolution of periodontal disease. *Where pockets are deeper however it may prove impossible for the patient to remove plaque deposits from the apical portion of the lesions, consequently some of the symptoms persist. The presence of bleeding from a pocket on probing indicates that there is residual inflammation. If there is no improvement at subsequent assessments pocket elimination procedures are indicated so that the patient can be given access to clean the root surfaces involved.*

Indications for subgingival curettage

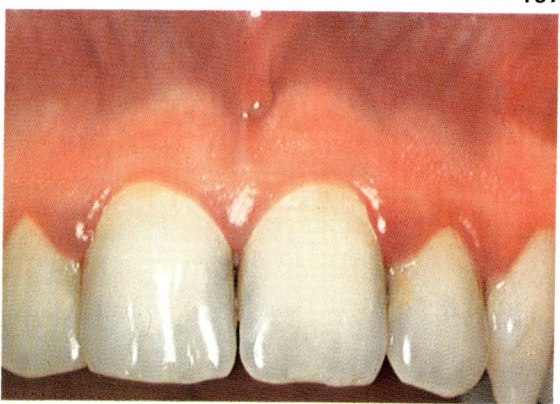

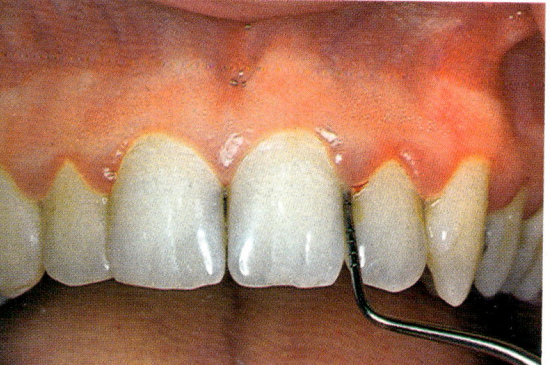

137. This patient has been receiving oral hygiene instruction and scaling over the previous two months. In spite of good plaque control there is still a persistence of oedema and erythema.

138. There are 3–4mm pockets interproximally and there is bleeding from the pockets on probing. It has been decided to use subgingival curettage to eliminate these pockets. This is a conservative surgical procedure which provides a maximum potential for reattachment (Ramfjord *et al* 1968). *Subgingival curettage is applicable where there are coronal pockets caused by oedema fluid, and shallow radicular pockets provided there are no infra-bony defects.*

Operative technique

139. The procedure involves the removal of the epithelial lining of the pocket and the epithelial attachment at the pocket base. The root of the tooth is scaled to remove deposits and lightly planed to remove cementum which may be contaminated with irritants including endotoxins (Aleo *et al* 1974).

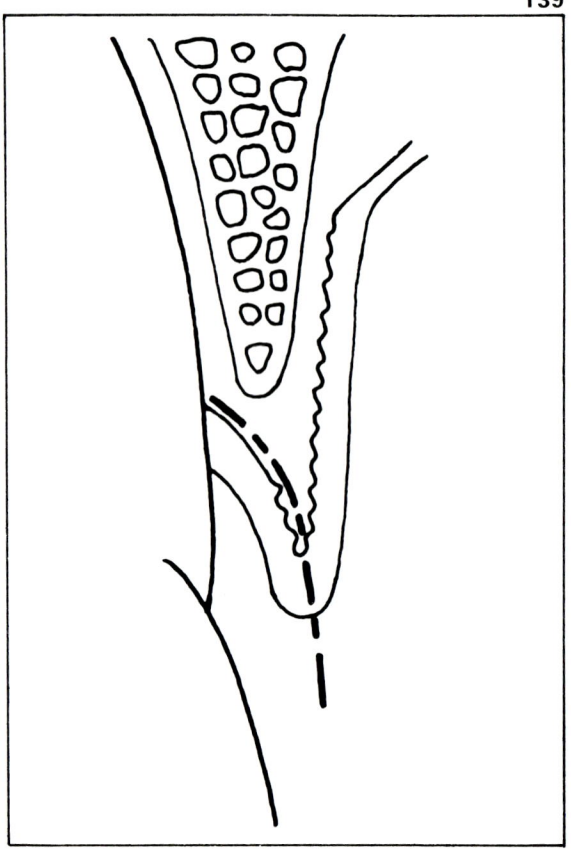

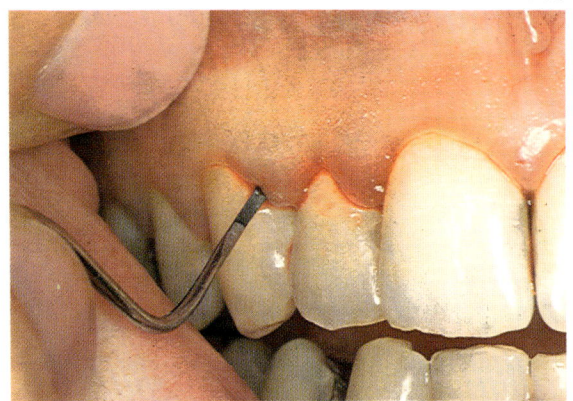

140. A sharp curette is being used to remove the epithelium from the pocket. The unsupported gingival tissue may be stabilised against the blade of the curette by applying finger pressure against the outer aspect of the gingivae.

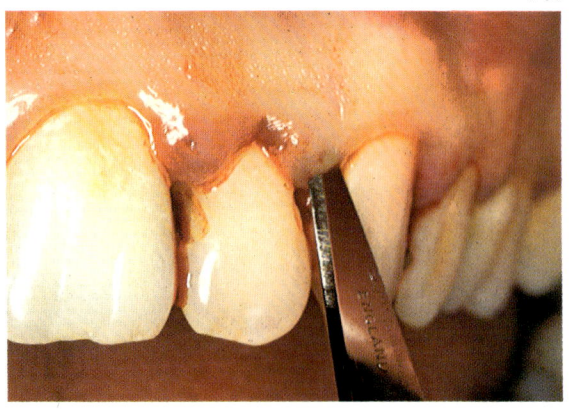

141. Curettage may also be performed by sharp dissection with a scalpel, this enables the line of the incision to be designed with greater precision. This is virtually the same incision as the inverse bevel (see Chapter 12).

Operative technique

142. Using the incisional technique the prospects of removing all the epithelium from the pocket by subsequent curettage are improved. Following curettage pressure is applied to the soft tissues to adapt them to the tooth surfaces. Sutures or dressings are usually unnecessary.

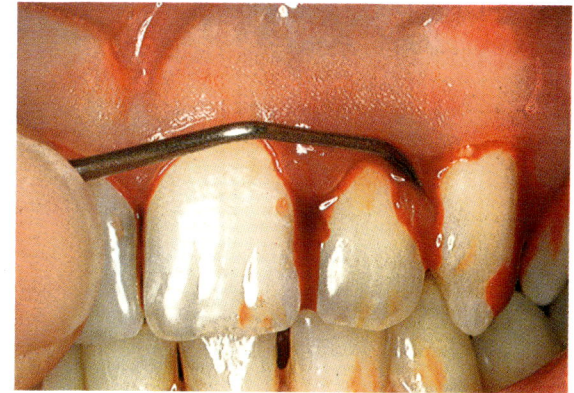

143. Three weeks after surgery the pockets have been eliminated and there has been resolution of inflammation. The reduction in pockets with this procedure is caused by a combination of recession of the marginal gingivae, reattachment of the junctional epithelium and regeneration of the periodontium (Chase 1974).

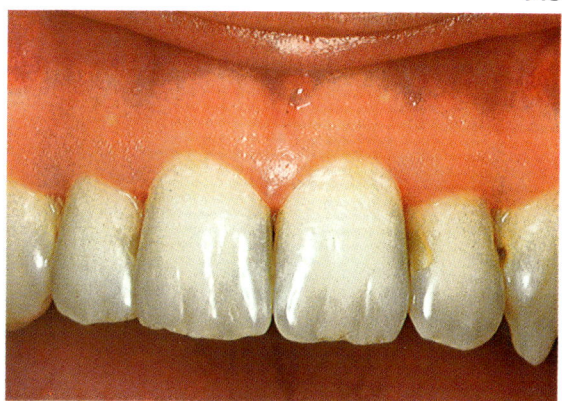

Applications of the procedure

Subgingival curettage imposes relatively minor surgical trauma to the tissues (Stone *et al* 1965). It may therefore be the treatment of choice for elderly patients, and for those with medical histories which preclude more elaborate surgical procedures. Where postoperative recession is undesirable because of aesthetic considerations, curettage may be used to reduce the inflammation without complete elimination of the pocket. The presence of a complex infra-bony defect may prevent the complete elimination of pocketing by periodontal surgery. If there is evidence of inflammation in a residual pocket after surgery this may be treated by subgingival curettage which can be repeated at intervals, when for example one finds that there is a recurrence of bleeding from the pocket on probing (Chase 1974).

11. The gingivectomy procedure

144 & 145. The rationale for periodontal surgery has been discussed in Chapter 10. The objectives of the gingivectomy procedure are to eliminate pockets by excising the unsupported soft tissue walls and to contour the gingival tissues by the technique of gingivoplasty to produce a physiological form which can be maintained by the patient. *The procedure may be used for the treatment of both coronal and radicular pockets* (**31, 32**). It should be used in preference to subgingival curettage for the elimination of gingival enlargement when this comprises mainly fibrous tissue. *Gingivectomy has a limited application however as it is contraindicated where there are pockets extending beyond the mucogingival junction, or where there are infra-bony defects* (**160, 161**) (Waite 1975).

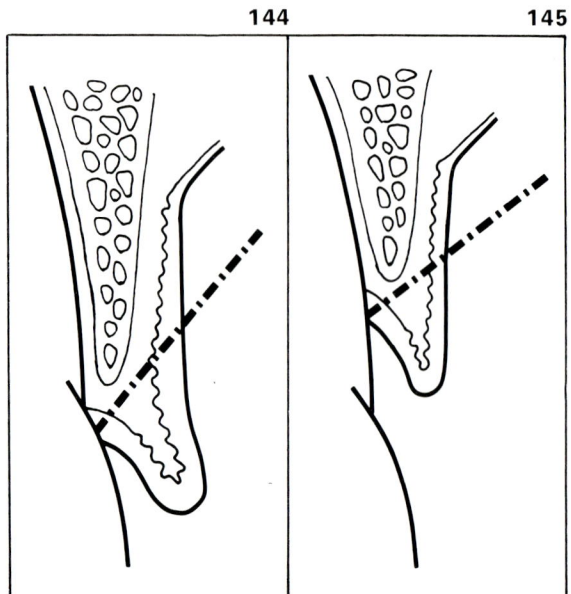

Operative technique

146. This patient has completed the oral hygiene phase of treatment. In spite of excellent plaque control there is still some enlargement of the gingiva resulting in coronal pockets with bleeding from the pockets on probing. The consistency of the gingiva can be assessed by laying a periodontal probe against the tissue and applying pressure; if pitting of the gingiva results there is oedema fluid present. Pocketing caused by oedema fluid may resolve with continuance of plaque control.

In this patient the gingival tissue is firm, indicating that it is mainly composed of fibrous tissue. Periodontal surgery is therefore necessary to achieve elimination of these pockets.

147. The radiograph demonstrates that there has been no interproximal bone loss which confirms the diagnosis of coronal pocketing. In other words there is gingivitis as opposed to periodontitis.

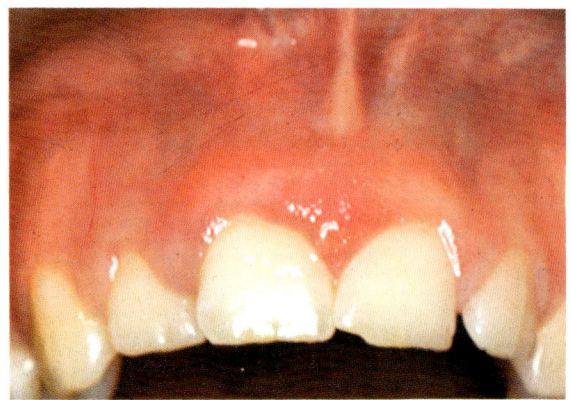

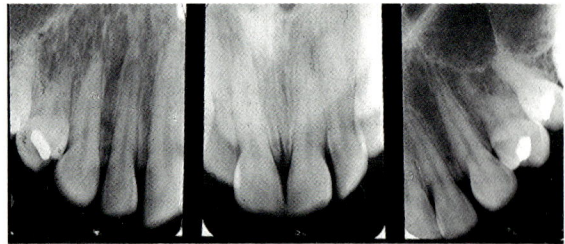

The gingivectomy procedure

148. Topical analgesic has been applied at the injection sites. Local infiltration of 2 per cent lignocaine with adrenaline 1 in 80,000 is being administered (see Appendix 6). For the labial infiltration the initial injection is made into the submucosa of the vestibule and the needle is then passed horizontally through the tissues at the level of the apices of the teeth. The solution is injected slowly ahead of the needle. Using this technique multiple infiltration injections are avoided. On the palatal aspect local infiltrations are made according to which area is being treated. In some areas nerve-block analgesia may be used but subsequently there is greater blood loss than when local infiltration techniques are employed (Hecht and App 1974).

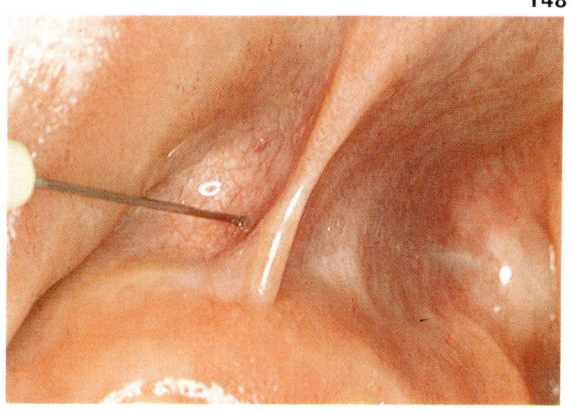

149. Additional infiltrations are then injected into the papillae and marginal gingivae. This results in further vasoconstriction and improved visibility during surgery.

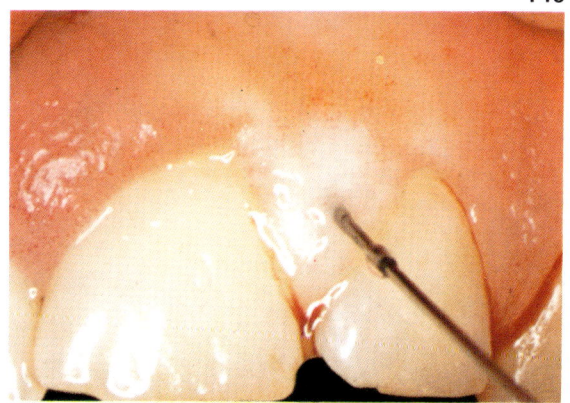

150. Pockets are measured with a periodontal probe and this measurement is transferred to the outer aspect of the gingiva, where the probe is up-ended and a mark made with the tip of the instrument.

An alternative method is to use pocket marking forceps; however these are difficult to apply interproximally.

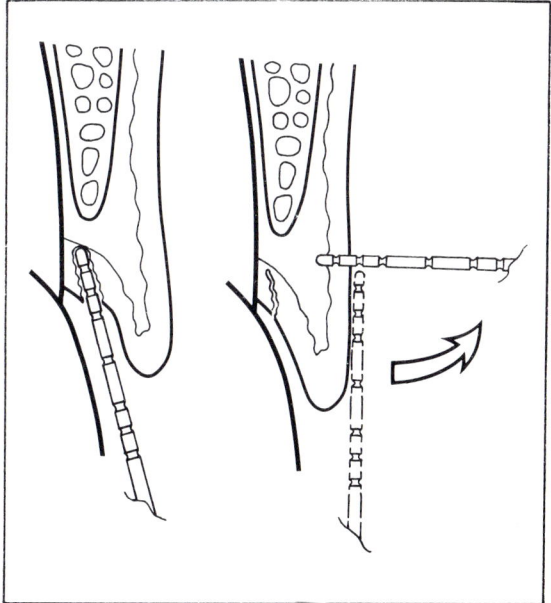

The gingivectomy procedure

151. The gingivectomy incision is commenced at a papilla, and is made at a level of about 2–4mm apically to the bleeding points which mark the base of the pocket. The position of the incision is determined by the thickness of the tissue and is designed so that a tapered margin will be achieved (Goldman 1951). The instrument being used for this procedure is the Blake gingivectomy knife. This has the advantage that it offers a sharp disposable blade which can be renewed during the operation if necessary.

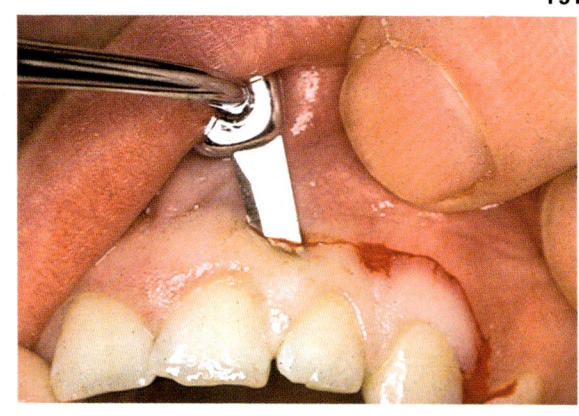

152. After the outlining incision has been made a tapered blade is used to carry the incision interproximally. The incision should be made from the back of the mouth towards the midline as this gives better control of the instrument and maintains an unobscured view of the tissues ahead of the incision.

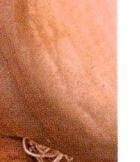

153. When the incisions have been completed the redundant gingival tissue is ready to be removed with a relatively heavy bladed instrument, for example a Cumine scaler or Prichard curette.

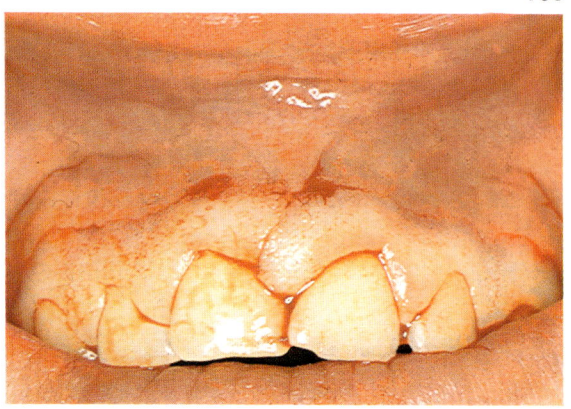

The gingivectomy procedure

154. The contour of the incision should be refined and blended with the outline of the intact tissue. The bevel of the incision can be enhanced if necessary at this stage. The contouring procedure, or gingivoplasty, is being performed with a scalpel using a scraping action.

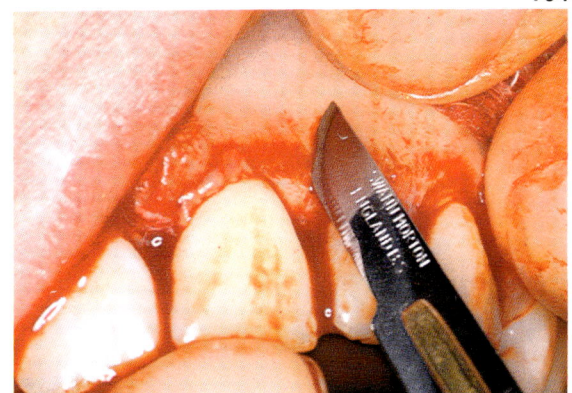

155. Alternatively the gingivae may be contoured using a handpiece with a diamond impregnated wheel under a saline spray.

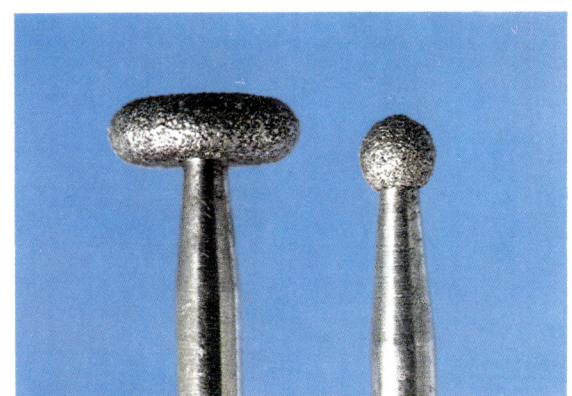

156. Epithelial tags and chronically inflamed connective tissues have been curetted away. The root surfaces have been scaled to remove any remaining deposits and have been planed until they are smooth.

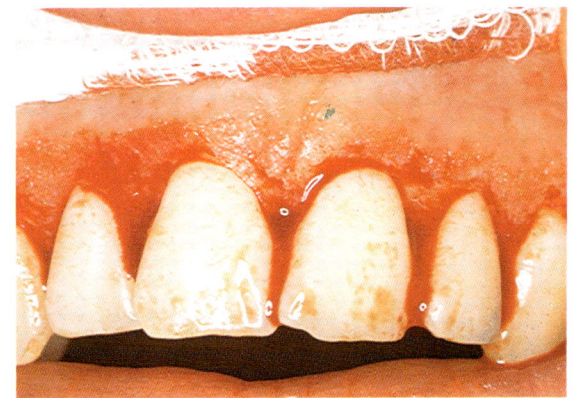

The gingivectomy procedure

157. A eugenol free periodontal dressing has been placed over the wound. This is to protect the area from trauma during healing and to reduce pain. The edges of the dressing must not be overextended. Pressure should be applied to the interproximal regions of the dressing with a cotton wool pledget covered with petroleum jelly, thus achieving adaptation of the dressing to the interdental spaces.

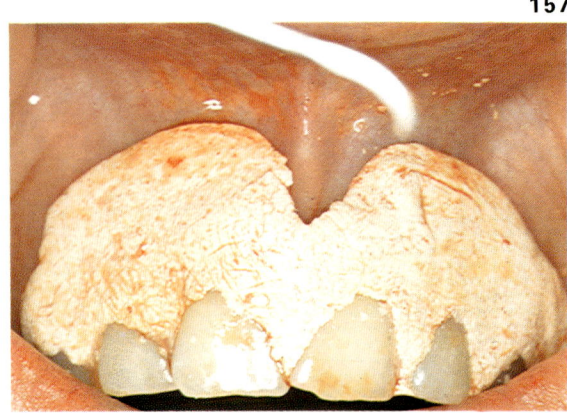

158. One week after surgery the dressings are removed and the teeth cleaned to remove residual dressing material and bacterial deposits. The epithelialisation of the wound has progressed well, but further maturation has to occur before healing is complete (see Appendix 10).

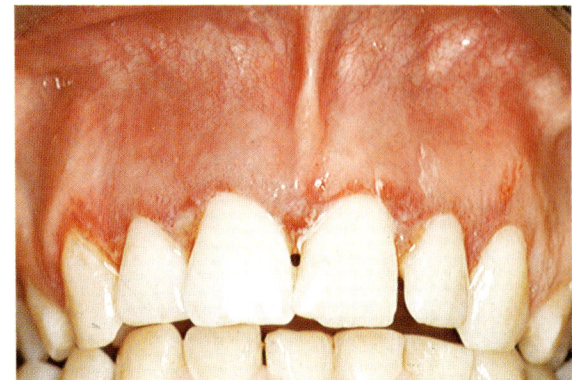

159. Six weeks after surgery there is satisfactory tissue contour, the pockets have been eliminated and there is no evidence of inflammation. The patient is maintaining excellent oral hygiene. It is mandatory that long term follow-up be maintained at regular intervals.

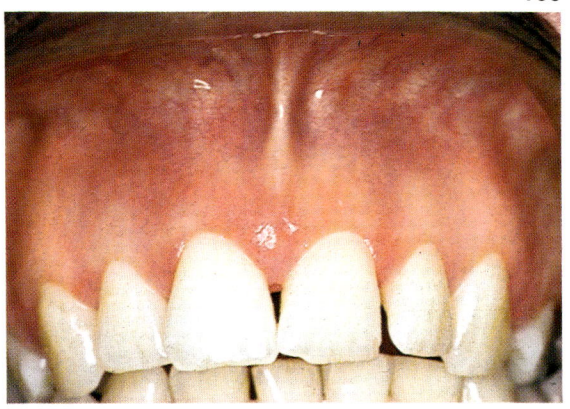

12. The inverse bevel periodontal flap procedure

Introduction

Indications for the inverse bevel flap procedure are as follows:

160. Where pockets extend apically to the muco-gingival junction, conventional gingivectomy would result in the excision of all the gingival tissue and is therefore contraindicated.

161. Where bone defects are present, the flap procedure provides good access for the treatment of osseous defects.

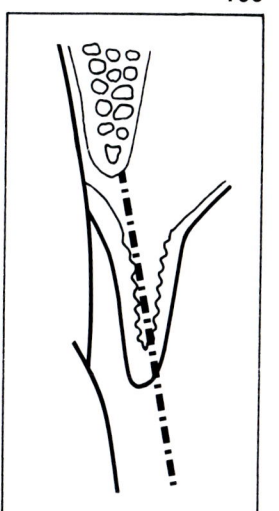
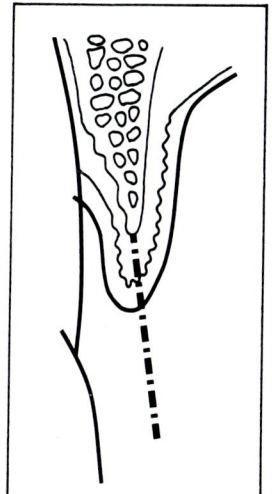

Operative technique

162. After completion of the plaque control phase of treatment this patient has residual interproximal pockets of 5mm. An inverse bevel flap procedure is indicated to eliminate these pockets, but at the same time it is required to conserve the maximum width of the existing labial and buccal keratinized gingiva as the pockets approach the level of the muco-gingival junction (Friedman 1962).

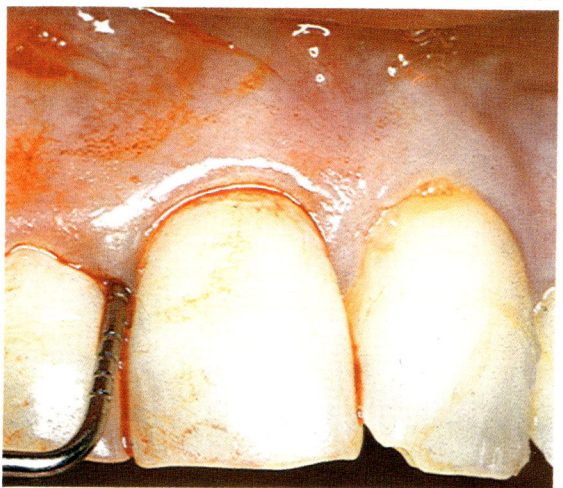

163. The region being treated has been infiltrated with analgesic. A vertical relieving incision is being used at the extremity of the operative site. This incision is not always required but may be used to improve access and facilitate repositioning of the flap. The relieving incision is commenced at the line angle of the tooth, where the papilla joins the marginal gingiva; adequate access is thus obtained for the treatment of the associated interproximal region. It is important not to position the incision on the marginal gingivae as this is liable to result in a notched outline after healing.

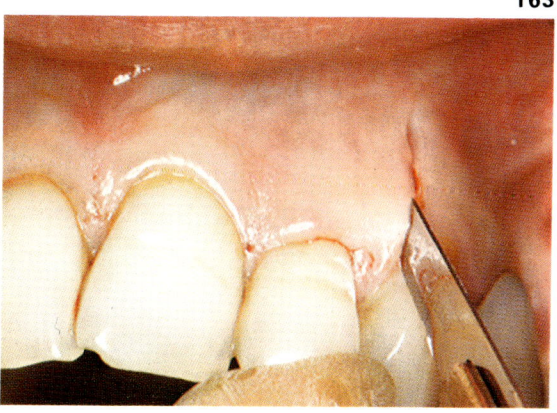

Operative technique

164. The inverse bevel incision is made with the blade at an angle of ten degrees to the long axes of the teeth and with a scalloped outline so that subsequently there will be adequate coverage of the interproximal bone. The incision should be made through the full thickness of the soft tissue to the underlying bone.

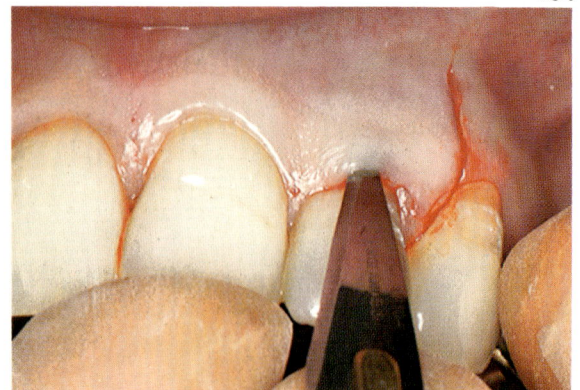

165. The flap is now elevated, the mucoperiosteum being separated from the bone by blunt dissection. Alternatively, sharp dissection may be used to leave a layer of periosteum covering the bone. The 'split-flap' procedure is only applicable where the gingivae are sufficiently thick to permit dissection and where osseous surgery is not required. Retention of the periosteum by this technique is indicated where there is dehiscence or fenestration of alveolar bone, or where the marginal bone is thin, making it imperative to minimise postsurgical bone resorption (Johnson 1976). See Appendix 10.

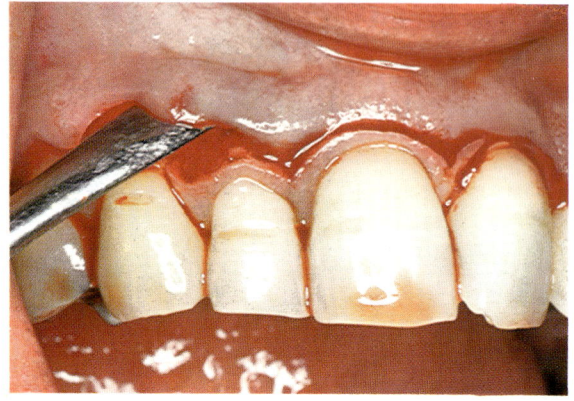

166. The flap has been elevated and the epithelium and hyperplastic corium which make up the pocket wall remain attached to the teeth. Prolonged inflammation has resulted in the proliferation of both blood vessels and connective tissue of the gingivae.

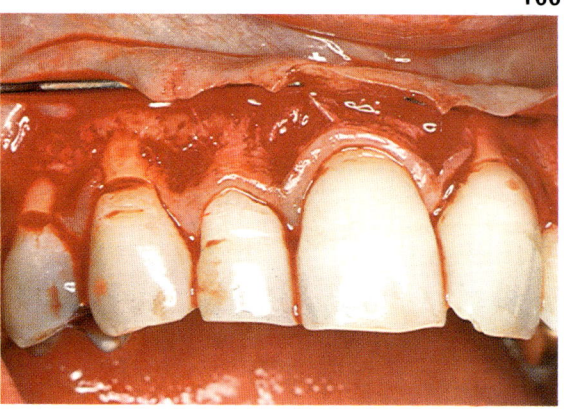

167. The redundant tissue is removed. Curettes are used to remove any tags of junctional epithelium, thus permitting the reattachment of new periodontal membrane fibres. Haemorrhage control is essential so that removal of all the hyperplastic tissue can be ensured.

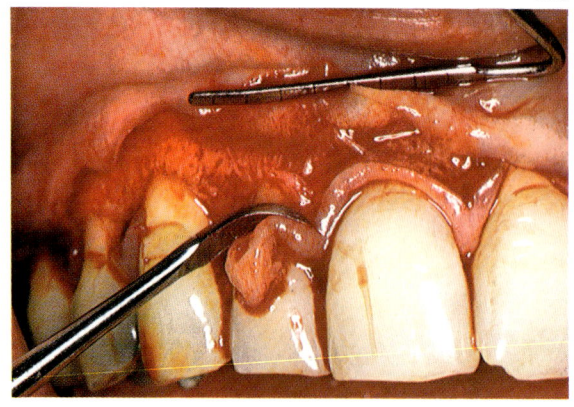

Operative technique

168. The root surfaces are planed and smoothed to remove retained irritants. A study by Aleo *et al* (1974) has shown that the cemental surfaces of periodontally involved teeth contain endotoxin; this finding reinforces the need to plane the roots of the teeth and to obtain smooth hard surfaces which are less likely to retain toxins, and thereby encourage reattachment.

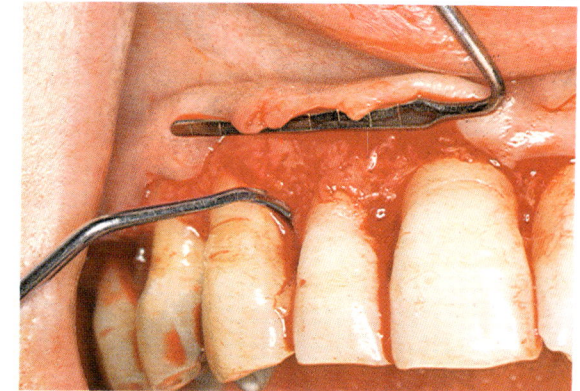

169. The bone contour is assessed; in this patient no osseous defects are present. Prior to suturing the field is washed with isotonic saline from a syringe to remove loose debris and irritants.

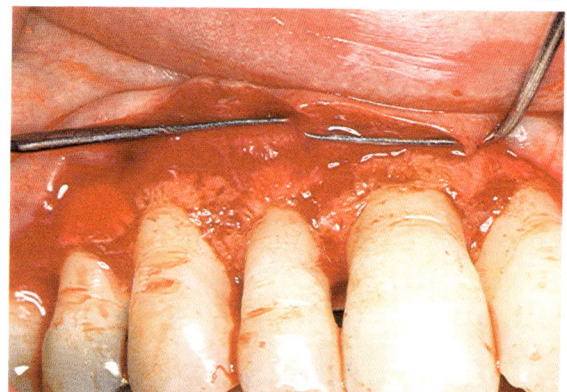

170. An inverse bevel flap procedure was used to eliminate the palatal pocketing and to remove the hyperplastic tissue (see **175**). This shows the palatal flap after curettage. Alternatively the gingivectomy procedure (Chapter 11) can be used on the palatal aspect, provided there are no infra-bony pockets.

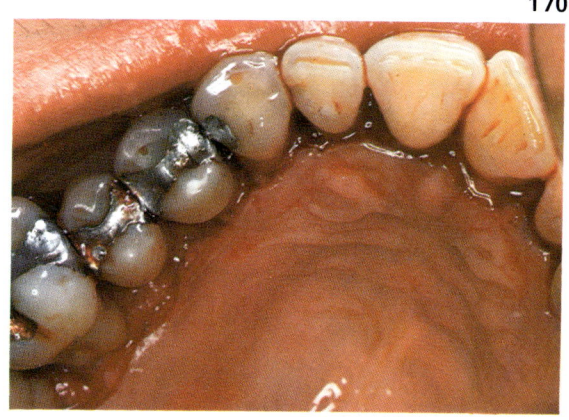

171. The placement of the flap prior to suturing is determined by several factors, which will be discussed subsequently. For this patient the flap is being repositioned apically by about 1–2mm. The flaps are held in the desired position by interrupted sutures; the tension is important as it determines the degree of apical repositioning. If the sutures are too loose excessive exposure of bone results, whereas if they are too tight the flap is pulled coronally onto the tooth surfaces. Where more radical repositioning is required the difference in tension between the buccal and palatal sutures may be achieved by using the continuous suturing technique (see Appendix 9).

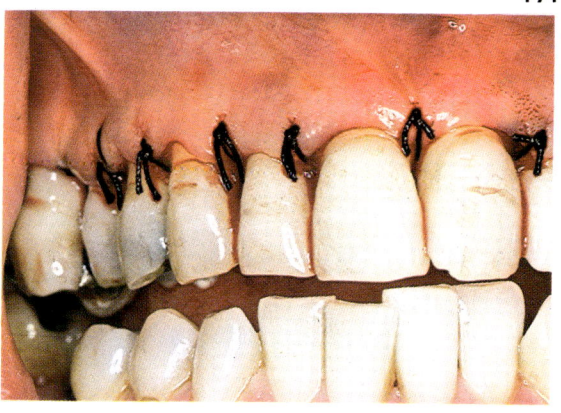

Operative technique

172. The placement of a dressing after flap surgery is not always necessary. Where the tissues have been repositioned the use of a dressing stabilises the flap. The dressing and sutures are removed after one week.

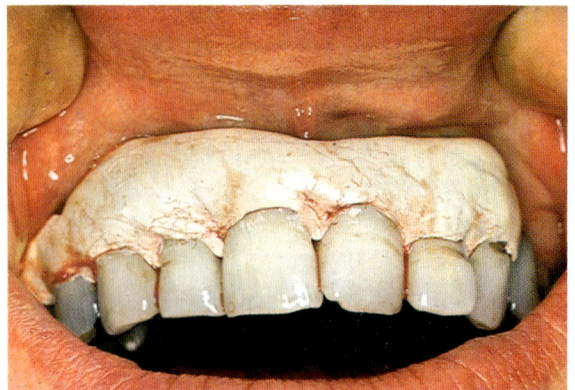

173. Six weeks after surgery a physiological tissue contour has been achieved. The patient has maintained a good standard of oral hygiene. Those areas where plaque deposits are not being removed should be shown to the patient and instruction given. The increased area of root surface exposed by surgery often causes initial problems, and cleaning and reinforcement of plaque control instruction is essential.

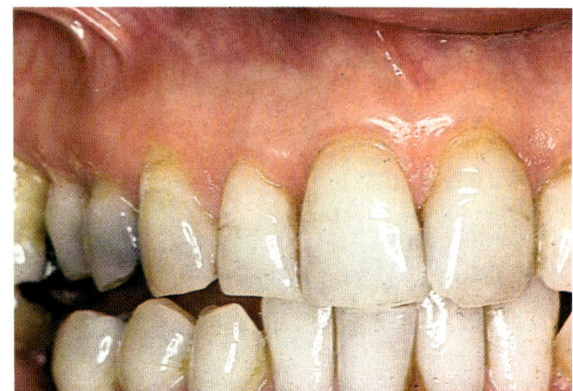

174. On the palatal aspect physiological form and sulcus depth have also been achieved.

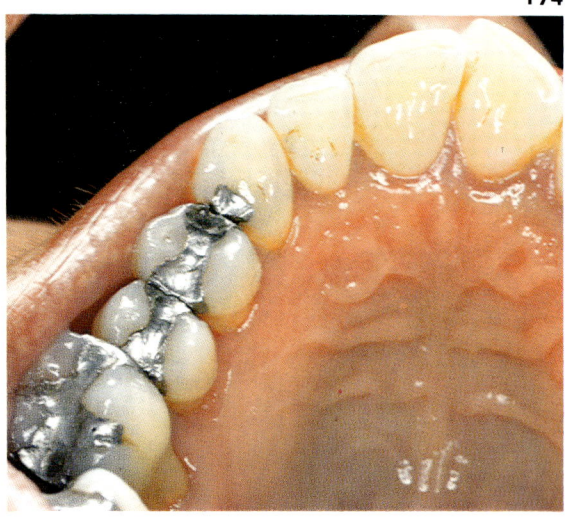

Modifications of the inverse bevel flap

175. The level at which the inverse bevel incision is made depends on the local anatomy and on the degree of periodontal destruction.

Buccal aspect
Where there is a limited width of gingiva as much of this tissue should be retained as possible. The incision is, therefore, made close to the gingival margin so that most of the keratinized tissue is conserved.

Palatal aspect
The palatal aspect is invested by keratinized gingival tissue which extends to the vault. This is relatively firmly bound down to the underlying periosteum so that it cannot be repositioned apically. Palatal pockets must therefore be eliminated by excision. The bone level is estimated by probing through the soft tissue at the base of the pocket. A mark is made on the outer aspect of the gingiva 2mm coronal to the level of the bone. The palatal incision is commenced at this level. If the tissue is thick it may be found easier to make the incision in two stages, an initial outline incision followed by a thinning incision. A longitudinal incision is then made within the sulcus to release the hyperplastic palatal tissue.

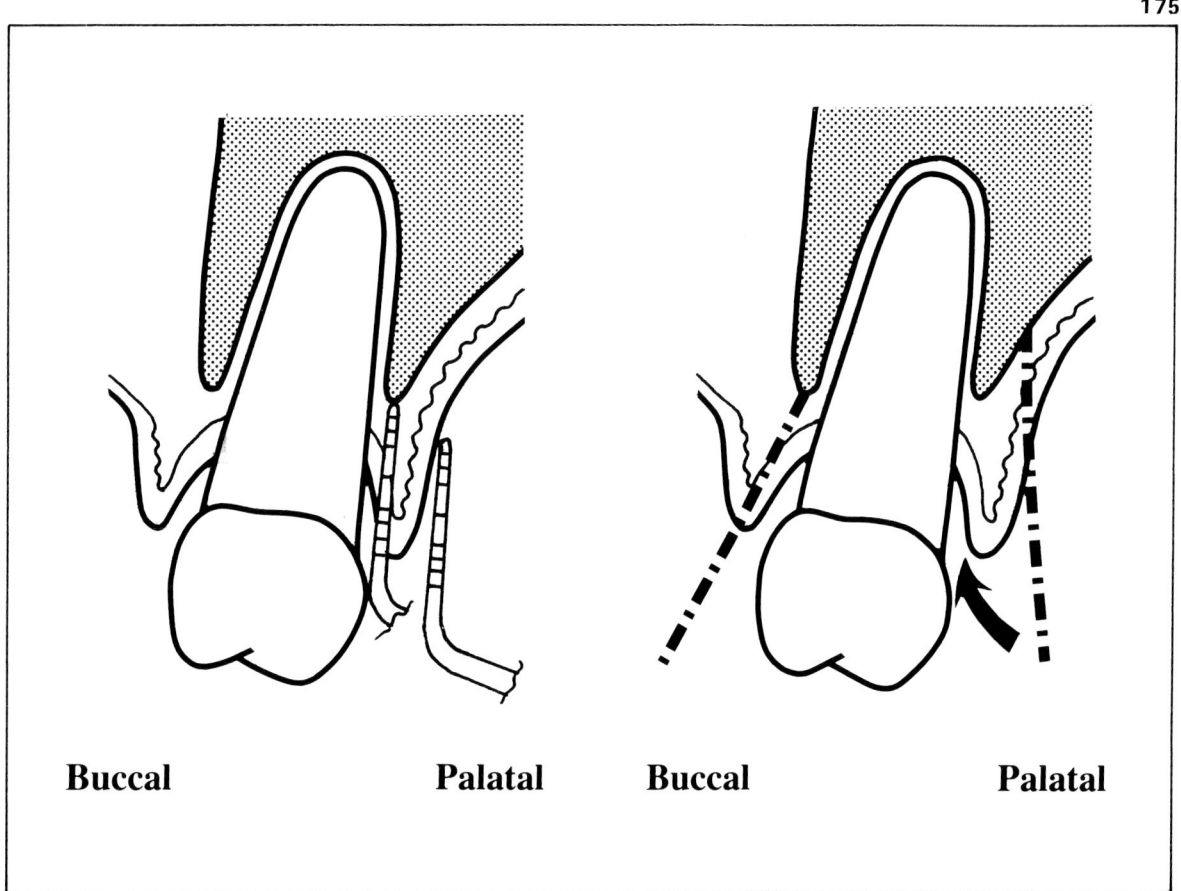

Modifications of the inverse bevel flap

176. The positioning of the flap prior to suturing has been mentioned earlier. This is determined by the following factors:

(a) If there is minimal bone loss the flap is replaced at the original level where it will reattach to alveolar bone. Under these circumstances the inverse bevel procedure offers an alternative to the conventional gingivectomy procedure for the elimination of false pockets.

(b) On the labial of the anterior segment cosmetic considerations may dictate that the flap be replaced onto the cemental surface of the teeth at the original level in spite of loss of bone. This procedure is not advocated routinely as attachment of the flap to cementum cannot be predicted. There is the likelihood of a downgrowth of epithelium and the formation of a long junctional epithelium, or possibly reformation of a pocket.

(c) On the palatal aspect the positioning of the inverse bevel incision is designed to result in the removal of the soft tissue wall of the pocket. The flap is replaced over the bone with minimal overlap onto the cemental surfaces of the teeth.

(d) Where there is established bone loss on the buccal aspect definitive elimination of pockets is obtained by repositioning the flap apically, which enables the existing keratinized gingiva to be conserved.

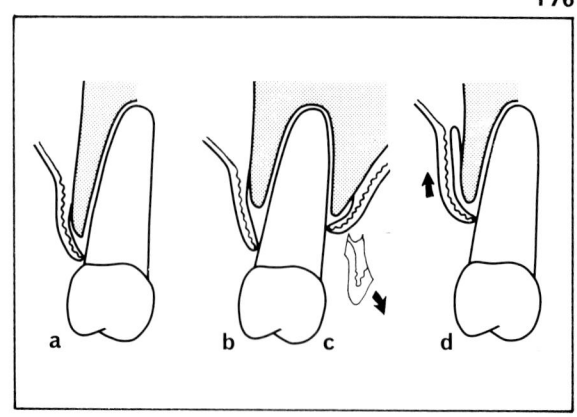

177. The inverse bevel incision may be extended to treat local pockets associated with the tuberosity and retromolar regions, and with edentulous ridges. The former are treated by removing a wedge of tissue distal to the terminal molar. The two incisions are made to be continuous with the buccal and lingual inverse bevel incisions. The width of this wedge is determined by the thickness of the tissue and the depth of the pocket. Following the removal of this wedge the flaps are thinned and where necessary trimmed to remove excess tissue. Pockets involving the edentulous ridge are treated by continuing the buccal and lingual inverse bevel incisions along the ridge. The two incisions are made some distance apart, this being determined by the depths of the pockets. When the central block of tissue has been removed the flaps are thinned and trimmed to produce an ideal contour of ridge.

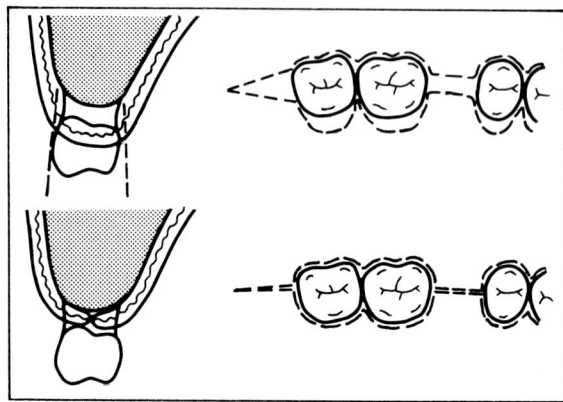

13. The treatment of osseous defects

Introduction

Where bone loss due to periodontal disease has occurred to an equal extent on each of the tooth surfaces, this is termed horizontal bone loss. In contrast periodontitis may result in bone defects of irregular configuration and this unevenness of bone loss may be caused by a variety of factors. The anatomical form of the tooth and variation in the accessibility of the surfaces to cleaning procedures may account for a difference in the concentration of plaque deposits, resulting in more severe periodontal destruction on one aspect of a tooth than on another. An additional cause of irregular bone loss is that the alveolus is not homogeneous in structure, being composed of the outer dense cortical bone and the inner trabeculated cancellous tissue. The cancellous bone is relatively vascular and is more susceptible to the destructive agents of periodontitis but also has a higher potential for regeneration.

A classification of alveolar bone defects is presented in Appendix 8. Osseous defects require to be treated at the time of periodontal surgery as they may prevent the attainment of correct gingival form, or they may result in residual pockets. Irregularities such as ledges or exostoses prevent the achievement of a tapered gingival margin, and infrabony defects are liable to cause recurrence of pocketing due to epithelial downgrowth into the defect during healing.

Osseous surgery

178. Where osseous surgery is to be used to improve the bone contour either rotary or hand operated instruments may be employed. Cross cut surgical burs are used at slow speed with a sterile saline spray as coolant. Burs are available for use in either straight or right-angle handpieces.

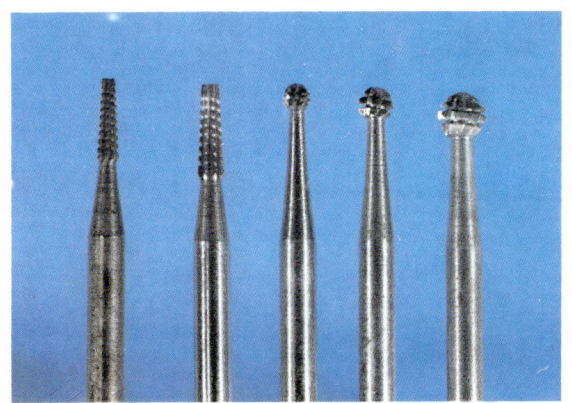

179. Chisels, such as the Ochsenbein instruments shown here, are used to contour bone in proximity to the root surface as there is less chance of damaging cementum when using hand instruments. Bone files are of value in achieving interproximal grooving. Hand instruments take longer to use than rotary instruments, particularly when contouring dense bone, but they provide greater accuracy.

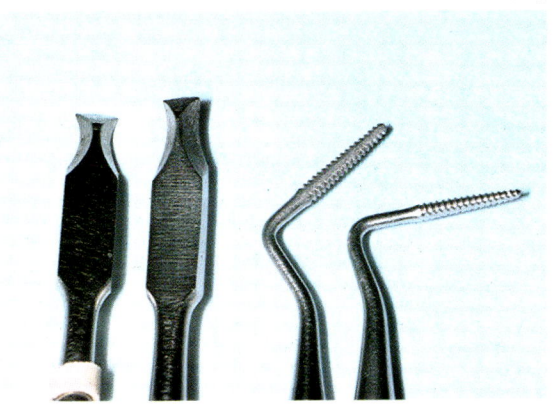

Osseous surgery

180. On this patient marginal bone ledges are being reduced and grooves are being established interproximally. The removal of non-supporting alveolar bone is termed osteoplasty.

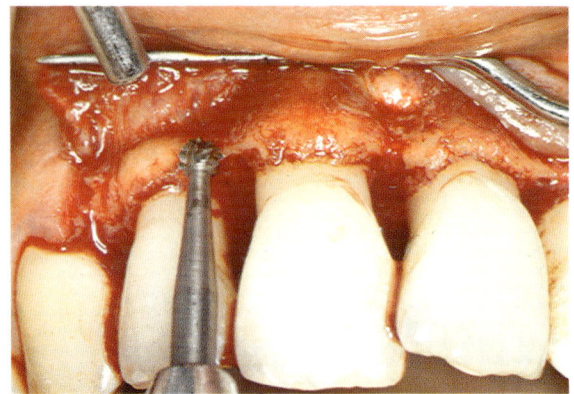

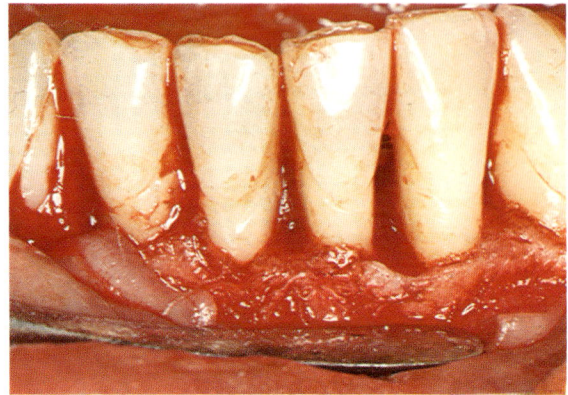

181. This patient has interproximal cratering and there is reverse architecture, that is the marginal bone is at a more coronal level than the interproximal bone.

182. The removal of some of the labial and lingual marginal bone is necessary to eliminate the craters and to reduce the degree of reverse architecture. The removal of supporting bone is termed ostectomy.

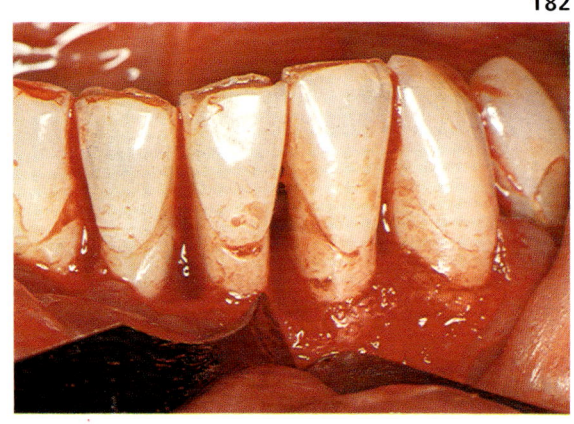

183. Bone removal has been performed conservatively. It is inevitable that the raising of a flap and the cutting of bone will result in surgical trauma to the bone with subsequent resorption and a further loss of about 0.5–1.0mm of marginal bone during healing (Wood *et al* 1972).

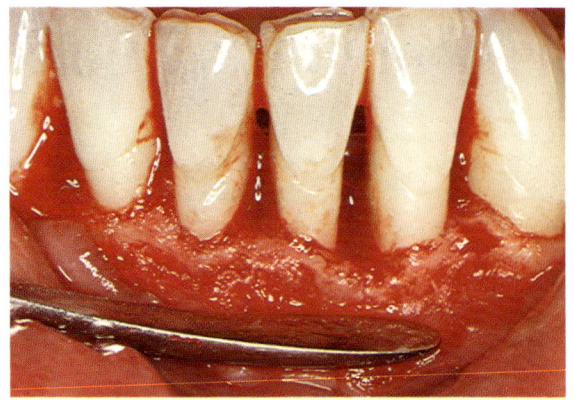

Osseous surgery

184. At eight weeks after surgery there is no pocketing present. However, the conservative use of bone surgery on this patient has resulted in a lack of scalloping in the gingival contour and a blunting of the interproximal papillae. This does not pose a hygiene problem to the well motivated patient, and the acceptance of this type of contour is recommended in preference to the use of radical ostectomy.

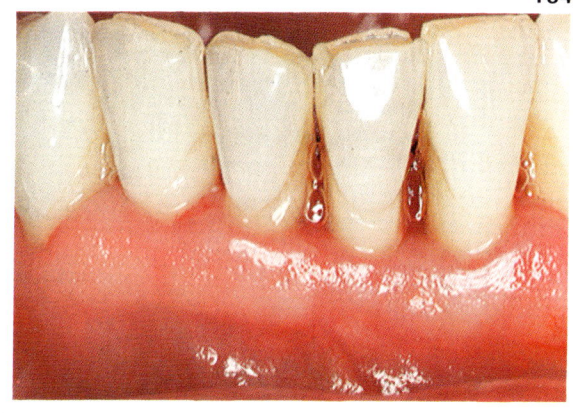

Regeneration procedure

185. One method of treating an infra-bony defect is by the regeneration procedure. This technique involves the curetting of all soft tissue from the osseous pockets. Access for this operation is usually obtained by means of the inverse bevel incision.

186. A blood clot is allowed to form in the defect and this is protected from the oral environment by suturing the flap under slight tension, and by careful application of a periodontal dressing.

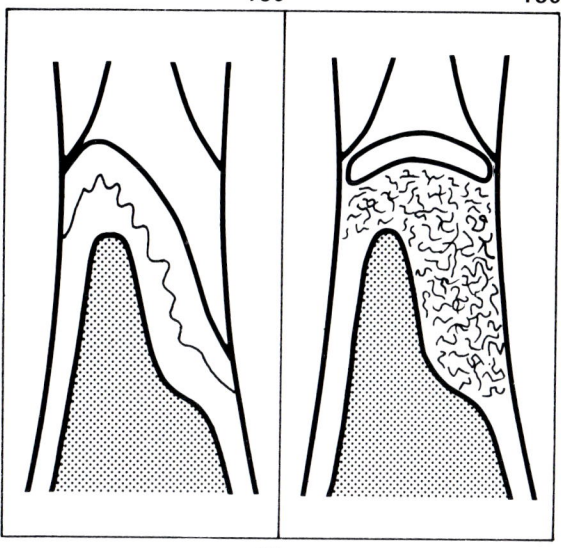

187. The objective of the procedure is to obtain a new attachment by the formation of bone, periodontal ligament and cementum in the bony pocket.

188. The achievement of this may be prevented by the downgrowth of epithelium into the defect which results in the reformation of a pocket.

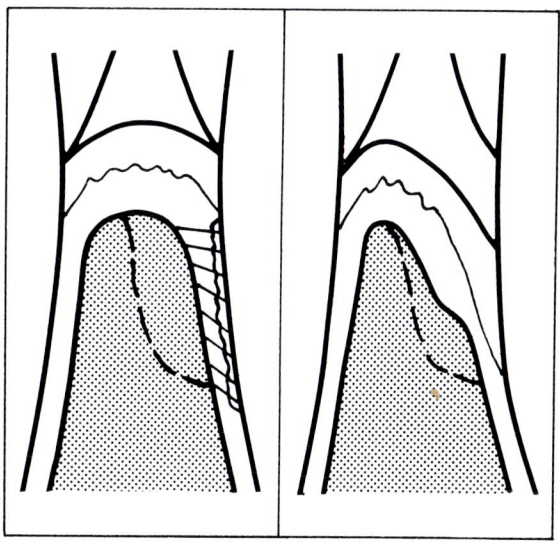

Regeneration procedure

189. A study by Ellegaard and Löe (1971) reported that three-wall pockets have a good prognosis for new attachment; over 72 per cent of the pockets in their study showed complete regeneration. Two-wall pockets were less successfully treated, only 45 per cent showing complete regeneration.

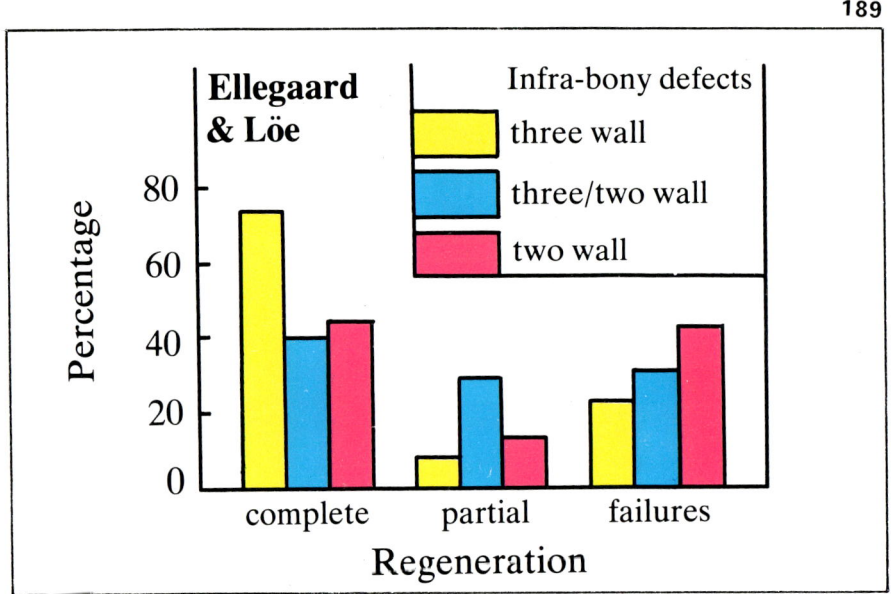

Grafting procedures

A variety of grafting materials have been used to fill bone defects after curettage, with the aim of preventing epithelial downgrowth. These have been reviewed by Ellegaard (1976). The characteristics of the ideal material are that it be accepted by the host with little or no immunological response, that it should enhance the osteogenetic processes of the host and that it should be replaced by new host bone. The most favourable results have been obtained by using autogenous bone. This may be obtained intra-orally from sites where osseous surgery is being performed, from edentulous ridges or from maxillary tuberosities. Cancellous bone is a better graft material than cortical bone as it presents a larger surface area for subsequent vascularisation and resorption. A number of studies have reported the successful use of autogenous hip marrow. This technique involves the patient in an additional, more major operation, and is only occasionally indicated. Its use might be justified when a large number of defects have to be treated in a highly motivated patient. The marrow should be stored by freezing before use, as fresh marrow has been shown to cause root resorption.

Other graft materials have been used with varying success; these have included allografts of collagen obtained from sclera and of freeze dried bone removed at necropsy. Xenografts of bovine bone which have been treated to modify the antigenic components have also been used. The main disadvantage of these materials appears to be that they are resorbed slowly.

Bone substitutes have also been used as grafts including plaster of paris and porous ceramic. These seem to result in delayed bone regeneration compared with other techniques.

Grafting procedures

190. This patient has completed a plaque control programme, but in spite of excellent oral hygiene there is still bleeding on probing at this interspace. Examination reveals the presence of a 5mm pocket confined to one papilla.

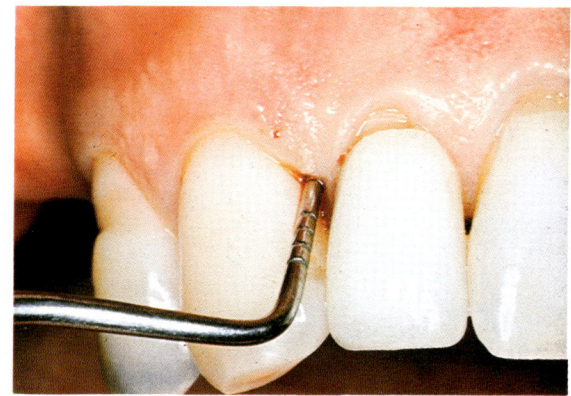

191. A silver point has been placed in the pocket so that the clinical depth of the pocket can be related to the radiographic bone level. There has been a loss of interproximal bone.

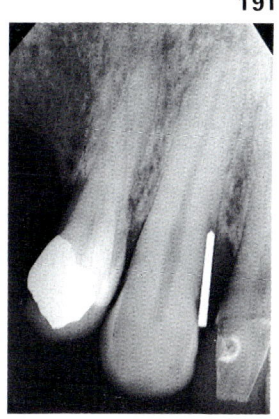

192. The raising of an inverse bevel flap reveals the presence of an interproximal crater. It has been decided that pocket elimination can best be achieved by means of a graft procedure, this being preferable to osseous surgery in view of aesthetic considerations.

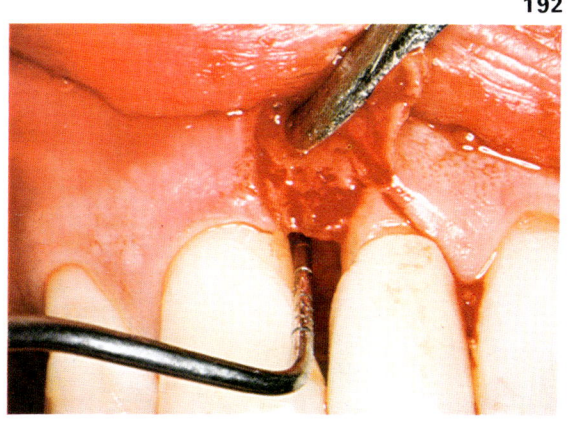

193. The bone is to be removed from an edentulous ridge area by means of a trephine which is used in a handpiece at slow speed with a saline spray.

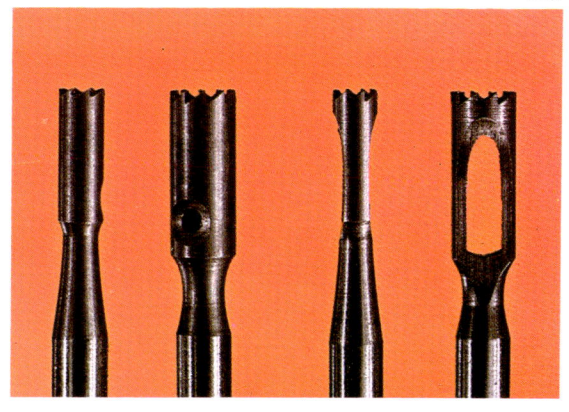

Grafting procedures

194. A core of bone has been outlined by the trephine and is ready for removal with a curette.

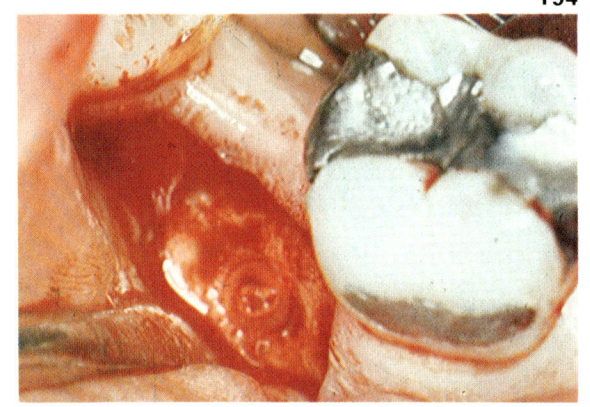

195. The bone has been cut into fragments and placed in the defect. A blood clot is allowed to form around the particles.

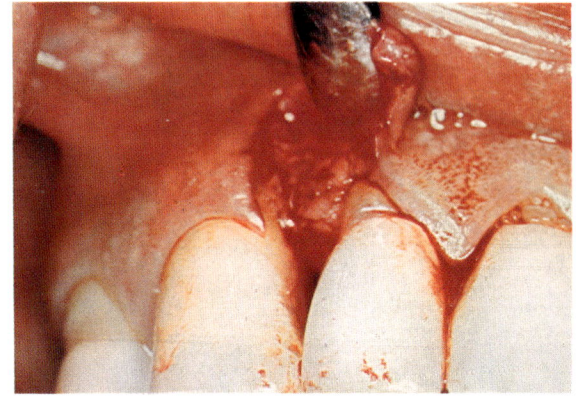

196. It is important to obtain good flap adaptation and following suturing a dressing is applied to protect the wound during healing.

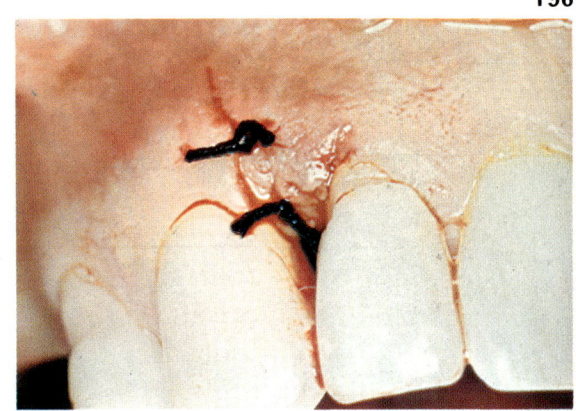

197. The radiograph indicates the level of attachment four weeks postoperatively.

198. At six months after surgery the grafted bone appears radiographically to have become more homogenous in texture.

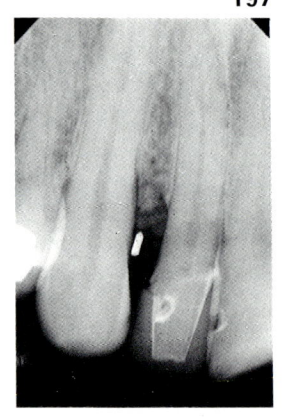
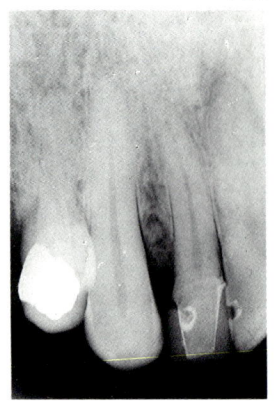

Grafting procedures

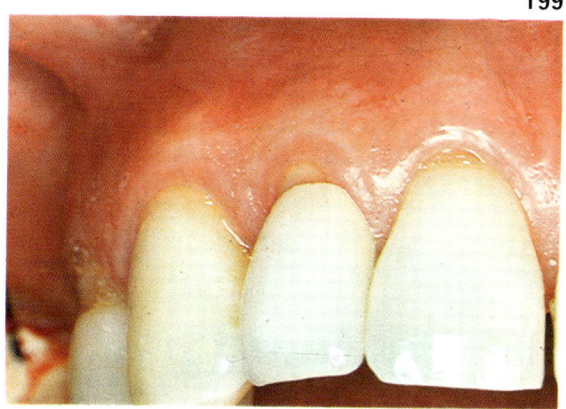

199. Clinically there is a physiological depth of sulcus and no bleeding on instrumentation.

Treatment of the furcation involvement

Multirooted teeth are liable to furcation involvement by periodontitis. Differentiation must be made between the furcation which has been exposed by the extension of periodontitis, and that which is involved in endodontic pathology via an accessary canal opening into the furcation region (see **314**). A diagnosis is made by probing for periodontal pockets and by testing the vitality of the involved tooth. Plaque removal by the patient from pockets which extend into the furcation region is impossible, because of the complex form of the root surfaces. The teeth at risk are the upper first premolar teeth, and the molar teeth in both arches.

There are several possible treatment techniques. Where the actual furcation is filled with bone but the approach grooves on either side are exposed, these should be thoroughly curetted and covered with a flap which has been contoured to provide a papilla-shaped extension over the groove.

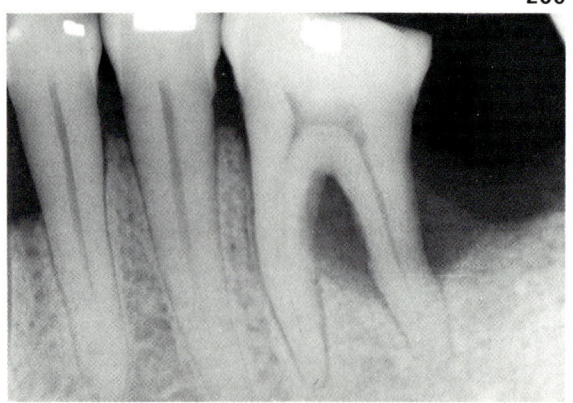

200. Where there is a wide U-shaped bifurcation this may be opened out by osteoplasty and by odontoplasty.

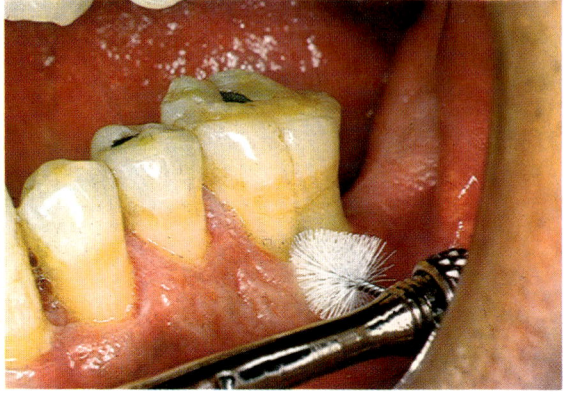

201. This is the clinical result after treatment. The furcation is accessible for cleaning by means of an interproximal brush. There tends to be a problem with the development of caries in the root surfaces after this procedure (Hamp *et al* 1975).

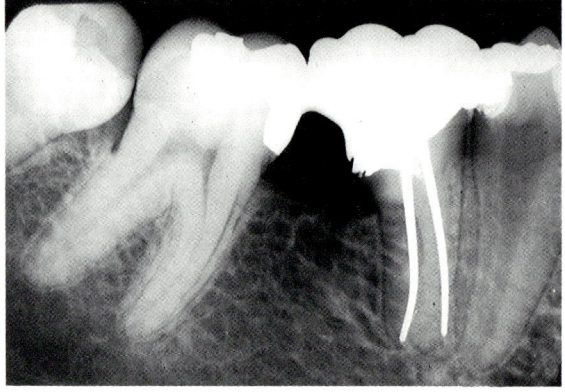

202. Alternative techniques include the amputation of one or more roots or the sectioning of a tooth. The bifurcation of this tooth had been exposed by bone loss. The distal root was more severely involved, and this has been amputated. As this procedure involves the patient in both endodontic treatment and periodontal surgery the extraction of the tooth should always be considered as an alternative, in relation to the treatment of the whole mouth.

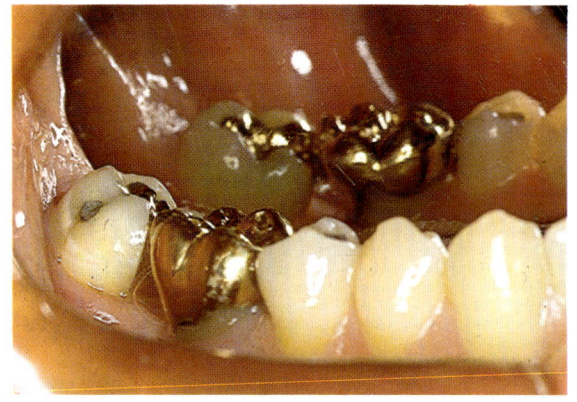

203. The previous site of the furcation and the crown of the tooth have been contoured to improve access for the removal of plaque.

The rôle of extraction

204. Where there is uneven bone loss and some of the teeth are severely involved by periodontal disease extraction of one or more teeth may be the treatment of choice.

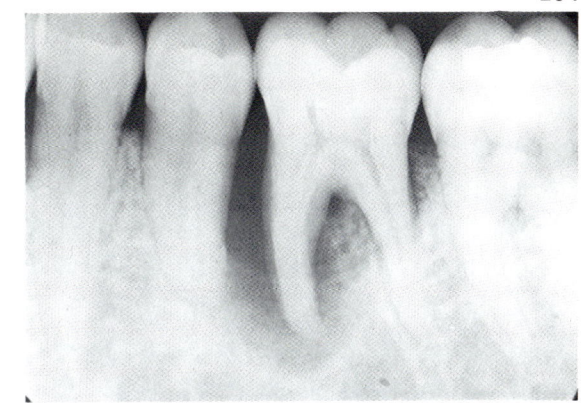

205. A radiograph of the same region one year later shows that the deposition of bone in the socket has resulted in the elimination of the bony defect.

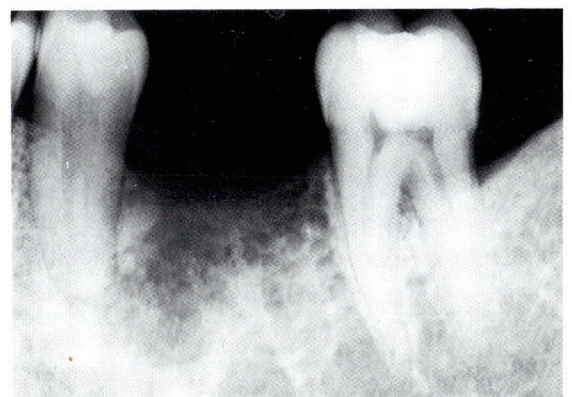

206. This patient has had periodontal flap surgery to eliminate pocketing. The upper right central incisor is very mobile (degree III) and the patient finds it causes discomfort when eating. During surgery and postoperatively a wire and acrylic splint had been used to stabilise this tooth. A disadvantage of using this type of appliance for prolonged periods can be seen on this patient, where caries has occurred as a result of leakage. The patient still finds that the mobility of the central incisor prevents his using it; a more permanent appliance is indicated.

When planning advanced restorative or prosthetic treatment the advisability of extracting severely involved teeth rather than splinting them should always be considered, as a reconstruction incorporating a tooth with severe bone loss may result in the early failure of the appliance.

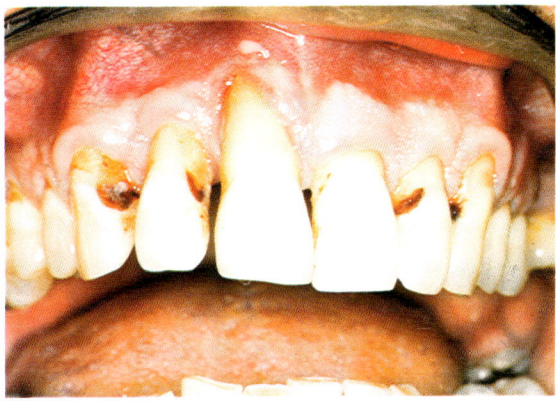

207. It was decided that the right central incisor had a very poor prognosis and it was therefore extracted. A stable result has been achieved by incorporating extraction in the treatment plan. In contrast if a fixed splint had been used to retain the central incisor the longevity of the appliance would have been restricted by the limited prognosis of this tooth as a result of the advanced bone loss.

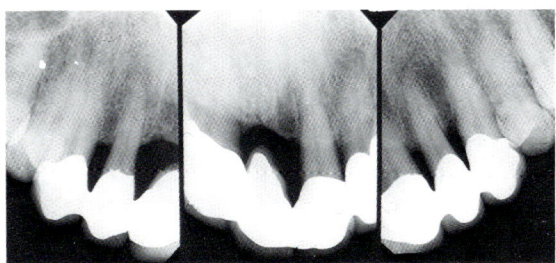

14. Frenectomy

Introduction

The objectives of the procedure are to eliminate a frenum and to create a zone of keratinized gingiva at the former site of insertion. Frenectomy is used mainly on the labial aspect of the upper and lower anterior regions but may also be used on the buccal segments and for the treatment of a lingual frenum.

Operative technique

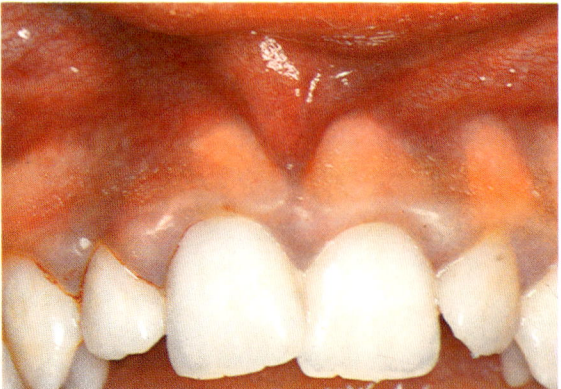

208. This patient has completed the plaque control phase of her treatment. On reassessment there is residual pocketing and the gingivae are still found to bleed on gentle probing. There is also a high frenal attachment which transgresses the zone of attached gingiva. The pocketing is to be eliminated by conventional gingivectomy.

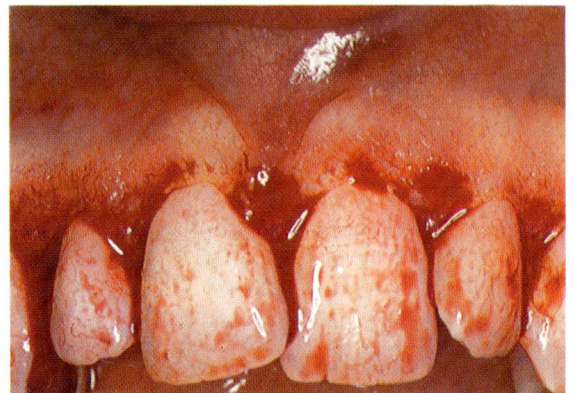

209. Following gingivectomy the influence of the frenum on the gingiva is assessed. Retraction of the lip causes slight eversion of the gingival margin, and it is considered that a frenectomy is indicated.

210. An initial V-shaped incision is made along the junction between the frenum and the gingiva.

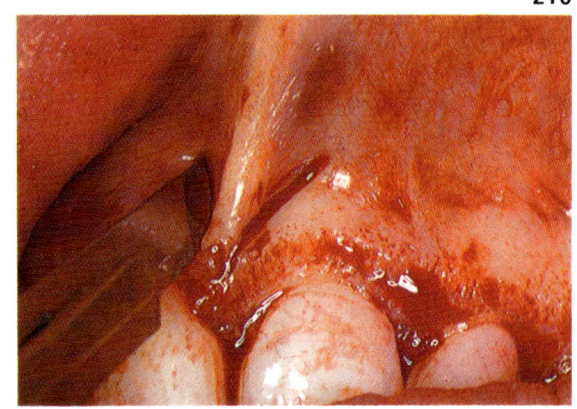

Operative technique

211. The frenum is grasped by a pair of artery forceps held parallel to the long axes of the teeth, the point of the forceps being at the level of the mucogingival junction. The frenum is then dissected free from the periosteum by an incision along one side of the forceps. An incision is then made along the other side of the forceps and the frenum removed.

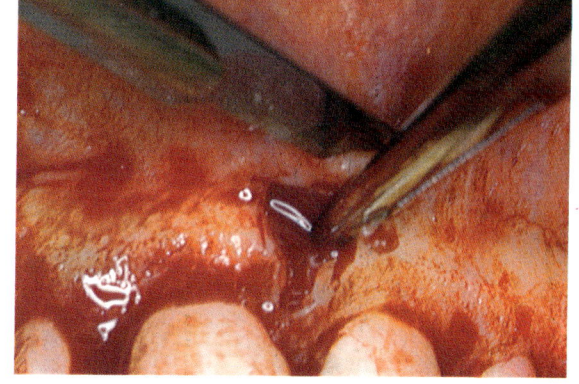

212. The periosteum is fenestrated at the level of the mucogingival junction to expose a strip of bone about 2mm wide. The objective of this is to produce a zone of gingival tissue which is firmly bound down to the underlying bone.

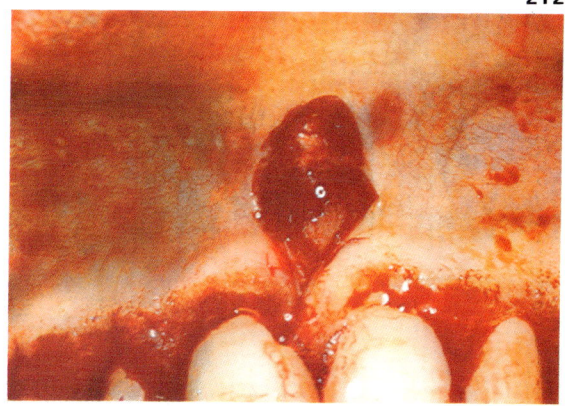

213. The labial mucosa is drawn together with one or two sutures, and a dressing is applied over the gingivectomy site.

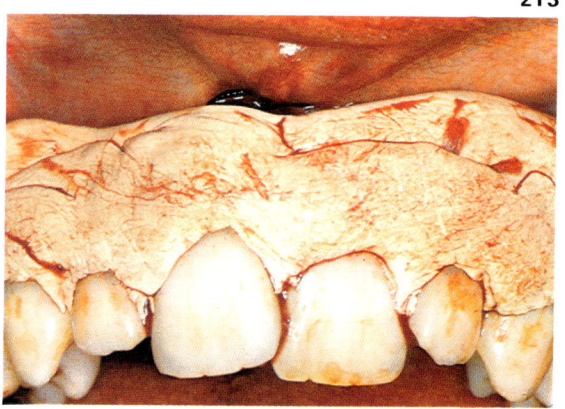

214. At two months after surgery healing is complete. A zone of keratinized gingival tissue has replaced the former frenal insertion.

A gingival graft may be used in conjunction with a frenectomy; this avoids the leaving of exposed bone to heal by granulation (see Chapter 15).

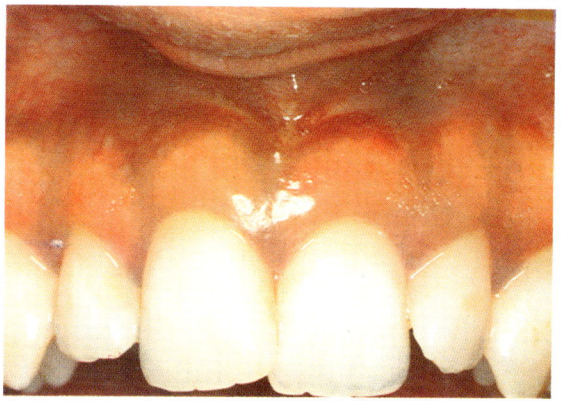

Applications of the procedure

215. This patient who is nine years of age has a high frenal insertion in the lower incisor region. The muscle action associated with lower lip movement causes eversion of the gingival margin which facilitates the accumulation of deposits; this has resulted in localised gingivitis.

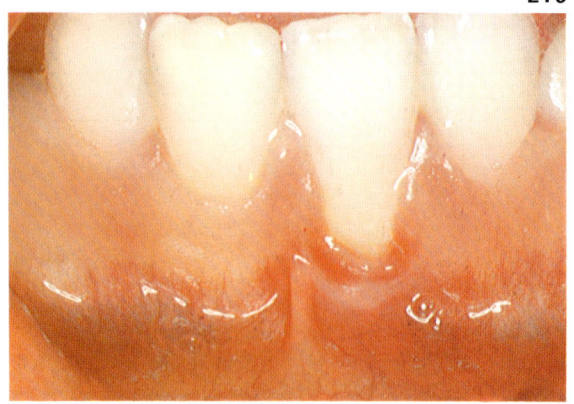

216. A frenectomy has been performed and there is a new zone of attached gingiva which prevents the transmission of muscle action to the marginal gingiva. The gingival tissue is now closely adapted to the teeth and the gingivitis has resolved.

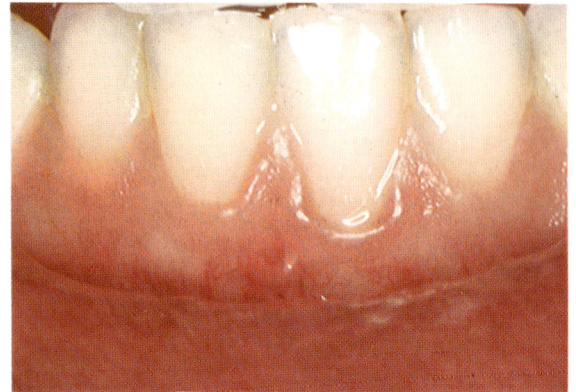

217. In this patient the large upper frenum is interfering with local plaque control procedures. Elsewhere in the mouth the patient is maintaining good oral hygiene.

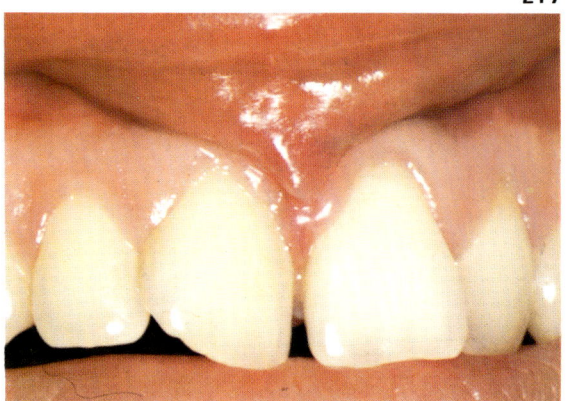

218. The frenum has been removed and there is now improved access for plaque removal.

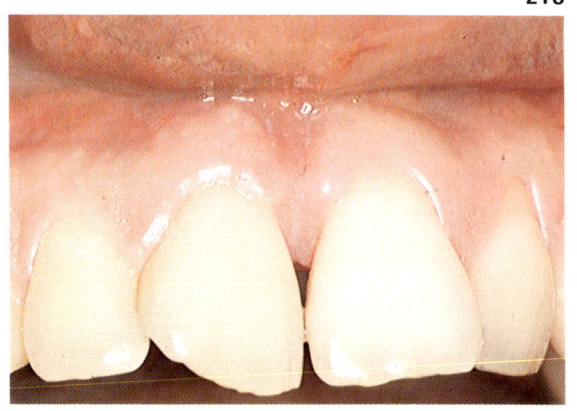

Applications of the procedure

219. When a midline space is present in the upper arch it is often found that the fibrous tissue of the frenum is continuous with the interproximal papilla. In these cases frenectomy is indicated and the surgical procedure should be extended interproximally to remove the band of fibrous tissue down to the bone.

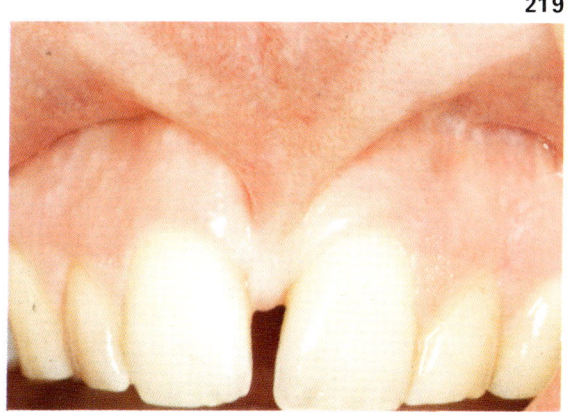

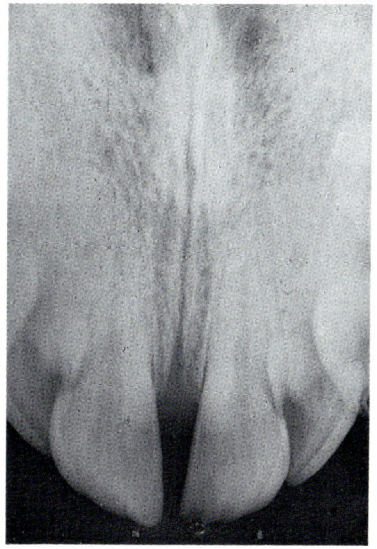

220. There is radiographic evidence of a wide midline fissure and at surgery this was found to be filled with fibrous tissue in continuity with that of the frenum.

221. For this patient removal of the connective tissue was followed by the gradual spontaneous approximation of the central incisors by mesial inclination of the teeth. Orthodontic treatment however is often necessary, particularly if the apices of the teeth are to be moved through bone rather than accepting approximation by tilting.

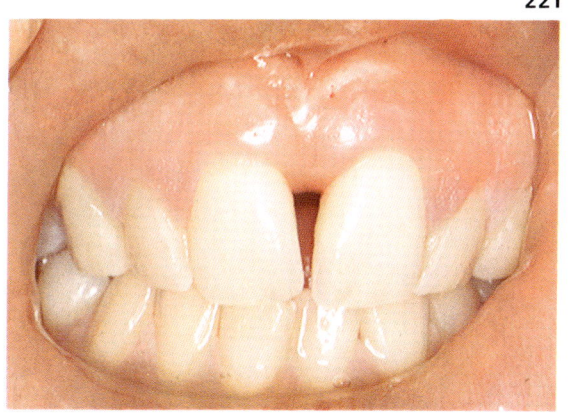

15. The gingival graft procedure

The gingival graft procedure is used to increase the width of keratinized gingiva. It may be applied to treat local pathology associated with an inadequate width of gingiva. The relationship between the width of keratinized gingiva and health is controversial (Lang and Löe 1972, and Miyasato *et al* 1977). Inflammation should be allowed to resolve after plaque control, and reassessment then made as to whether there are localised symptoms related to those areas where there are deficiencies in the width of gingival tissue. The indications for the free graft procedure following the plaque control phase are:

(1) To eliminate frenal activity when this is associated with persistent inflammation.

(2) As an adjunct to frenectomy where a high frenal attachment is hindering plaque removal with consequent local inflammation.

(3) To prevent the continuance of recession where this is associated with an inadequate width of keratinized gingiva.

(4) To reduce gingival recession on a tooth, using a coronally repositioned gingival graft. This procedure is relatively new, and long term results are not available.

(5) Preparatory to conservative procedures in which the margins are to be placed in proximity to the gingiva and where there is a minimal zone of keratinized gingiva.

222. The plaque control phase of treatment has been completed for this patient. There is a persistence of marginal inflammation on the lower central incisor evidenced by localised bleeding on probing. This is attributed to an absence of attached gingiva and an active labial frenum, causing retraction of the margin which aids the ingress of microorganisms. The gingival graft procedure is to be used to correct this lack of attached gingiva. Infiltration analgesia has been administered.

223. An incision is made along the mucogingival junction and sharp dissection is used to prepare the graft bed. The prognosis of the graft procedure is improved when a band of gingival tissue can be retained, thus creating a recipient site with a circumferential blood supply. The alveolar mucosa, muscle attachments and periosteum are displaced apically, exposing bone (Dordick *et al* 1976). It is important that the mucosal flap is made sufficiently mobile by dissection to prevent its subsequent encroachment onto the grafted area during healing.

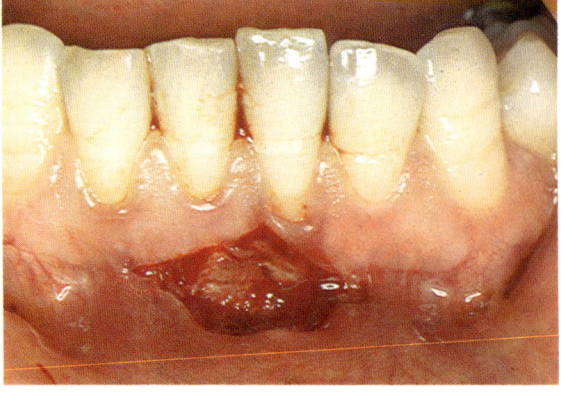

The gingival graft procedure

224. A tin-foil template of the prepared site may be made as a pattern for the graft.

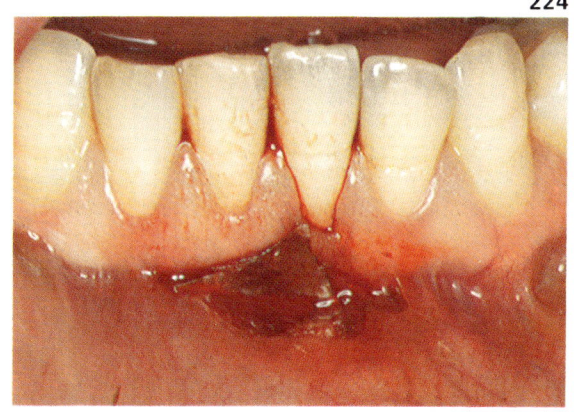

225. An appropriate donor site is selected. The most common site is the keratinized gingival tissue of the palate. The outline incision for the graft is made about 3mm away from the gingival margin. Commencing from the coronal edge a graft of about 1.5mm thickness is prepared by dissection, which incorporates some of the corium from the donor site (see Appendix 10, final section).

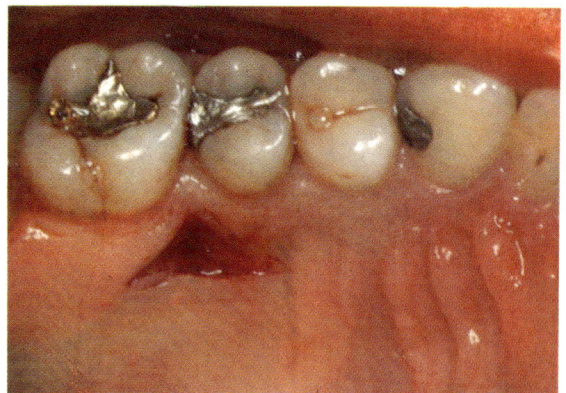

226. Following the preparation of the graft it should be transferred with as little delay as possible to the donor site.

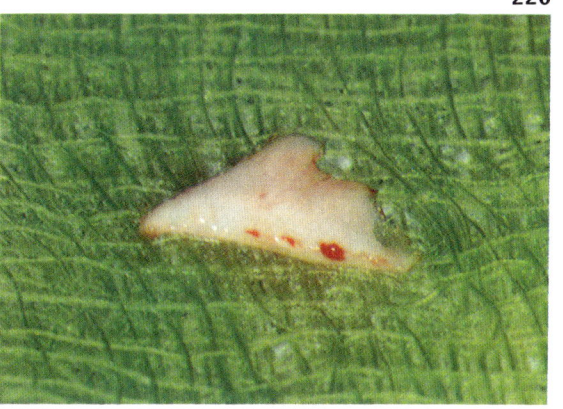

227. The graft is maintained in position by fine sutures (00000). These must not be placed under tension. Pressure is applied to the graft for five minutes to prevent the formation of a haematoma, and to promote the formation of an initial fibrin attachment, with the graft and donor site in close proximity (Sullivan and Atkins 1968).

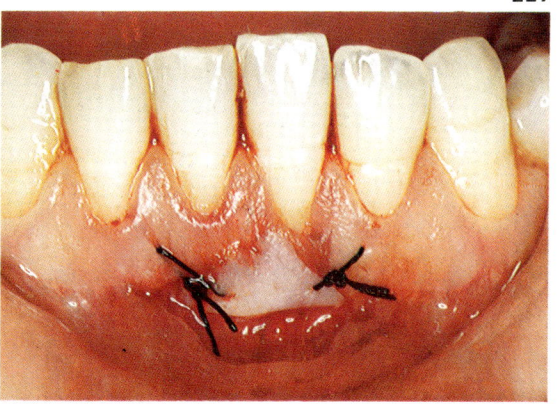

The gingival graft procedure

228. A dressing is placed over the grafted area. On the donor site stabilisation may prove difficult and a suture over the dressing may aid retention. For larger donor areas an acrylic palatal plate may be used to prevent the wound from being traumatised and to reduce pain.

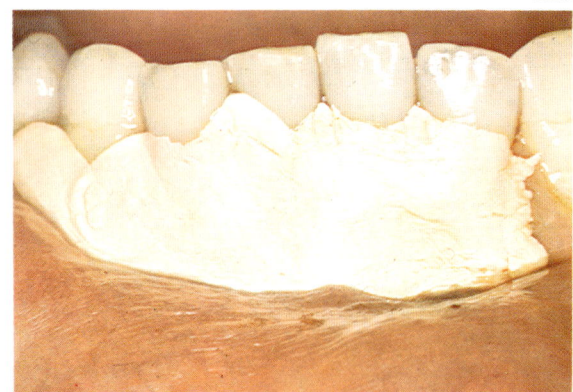

229. On removal of the dressing and sutures after one week, it can be seen that the superficial layers of epithelial cells have been shed from the grafted tissue. Attachment has been established between the corium of the graft and the recipient site. There is usually no need to apply another dressing. Instruction in postoperative oral hygiene is essential.

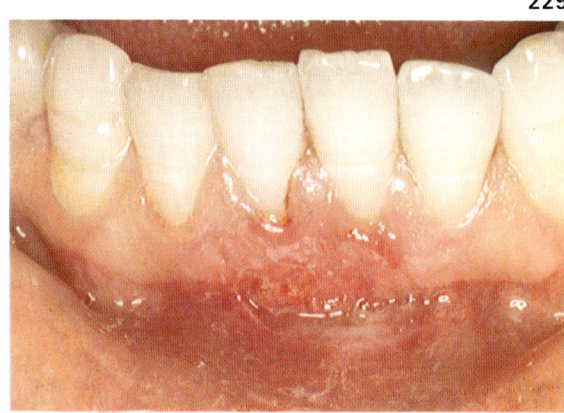

230. Eight weeks after surgery the grafted gingiva is paler than the surrounding tissue. This is often a permanent characteristic and may be due to an increased thickness of either the keratinized epithelium or the corium. There is a firm attachment of the graft to underlying bone. The effectiveness of the graft procedure was demonstrated by Ward (1974); he reported that the treatment of localised areas of recession resulted in a mean reattachment of junctional epithelium of 1.1mm, a reduction in pocketing by 0.4mm and a reduction in marginal recession of 0.7mm.

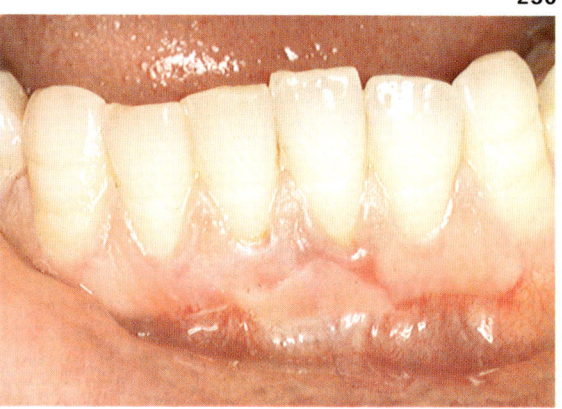

Application of the procedure

231. The gingival graft procedure has proved very useful for the treatment of large frenae as an adjunct to frenectomy as it avoids having to expose an extensive area of alveolar bone. A predetermined width of keratinized epithelium can be produced according to the size of graft placed. Surgery was indicated for this patient as the high frenal attachment was interfering with plaque control, even with the use of an interspace brush. Elsewhere in the mouth the patient had excellent oral hygiene.

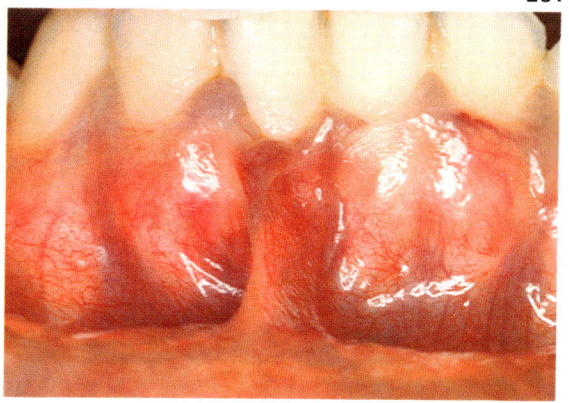

232. Eight months after surgery the gingival graft has healed well. There is now unrestricted access for plaque control and the patient is coping well with oral hygiene procedures throughout the mouth.

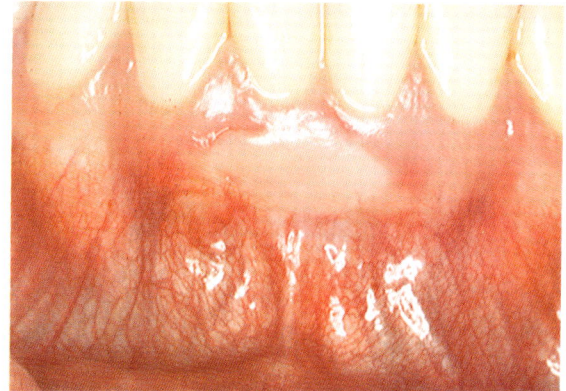

233. This patient has been under observation for over a year, and measurement of the level of the gingival margin in relation to the enamel cement junction has demonstrated that the recession on the lower premolar is still progressing. There is no keratinized gingiva on this tooth. The patient has maintained excellent oral hygiene throughout the course of treatment. There is a tendency for the mucosa on the premolar to become abraded by toothbrushing.

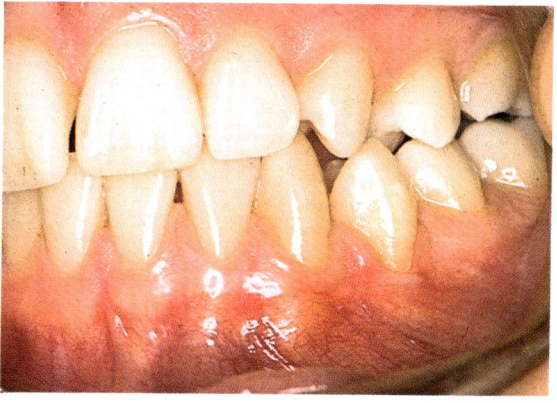

234. A zone of attached gingiva has been obtained on this tooth by means of a gingival graft. Follow-up assessment is indicated to ensure that stability of the gingival margin has been achieved.

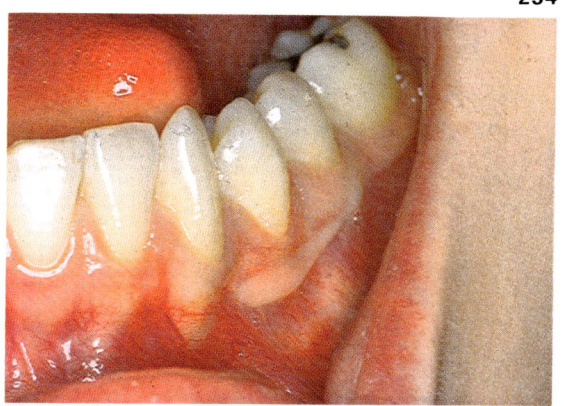

Application of the procedure

235. This patient has an Angle Class II div. ii occlusion.

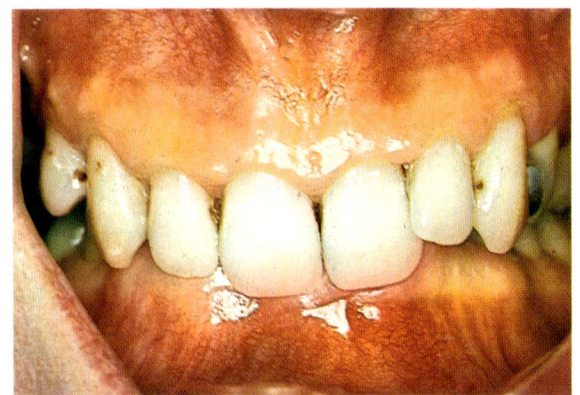

236. The upper anterior teeth are traumatising the lower labial soft tissues and this is causing recession. The trauma has resulted in the loss of the marginal attached gingiva on the lower incisor teeth.

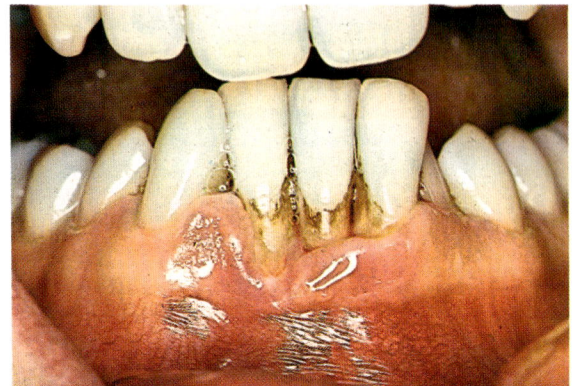

237. Following the plaque control phase of treatment a gingival graft has been placed to re-establish a zone of attached gingiva. The new gingival tissue is located further apically than the original marginal gingiva and in this position it is not subjected to trauma from the upper incisors.

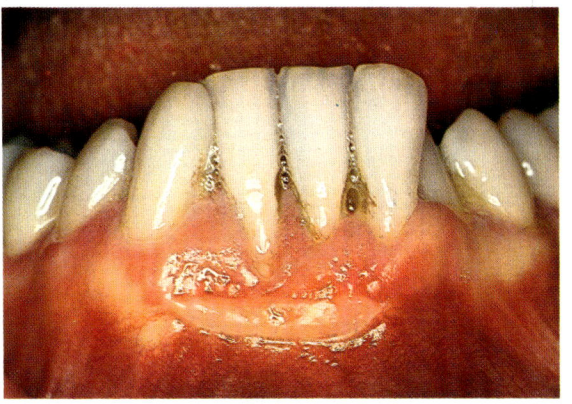

Application of the procedure

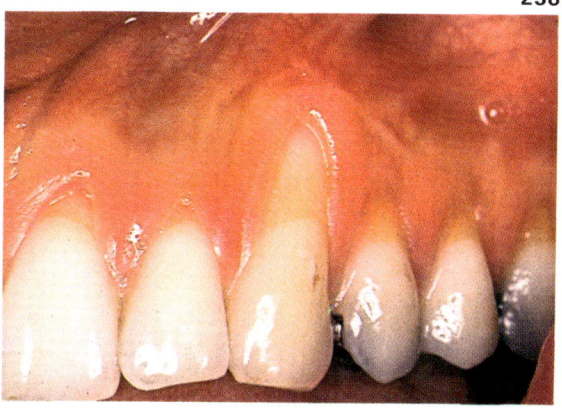

238. The treatment of localised recession by means of a gingival graft placed on cementum is unpredictable. The best prognosis is when the original defect is shallow and narrow, and the least favourable is when the defect is deep and wide, as here. The vitality of grafted gingiva is dependent on the proximity of the blood supply to that part of the graft which is over cementum (Sullivan and Atkins 1968).

This patient is concerned about the appearance of the recession on the upper canine tooth, which is visible when the patient smiles.

The recession will be treated by a two stage procedure. A gingival graft will first be placed on bone and two months later the grafted tissue will be moved coronally to cover the cementum, relieving incisions being used to release the tissue (Bernimoulin *et al* 1975).

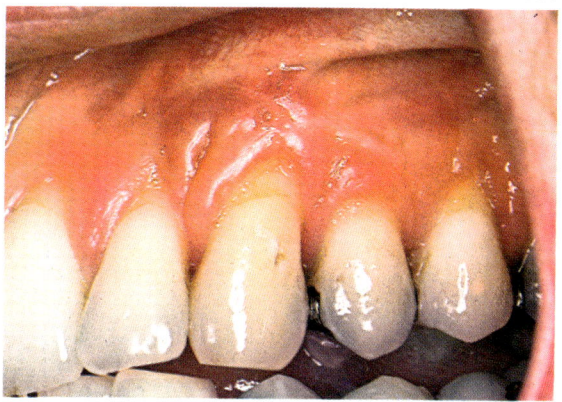

239. This shows the appearance four months after completion of the coronally repositioned gingival graft procedure. There has been considerable reduction of recession, however the patient has been warned about the uncertain long term prognosis of the procedures.

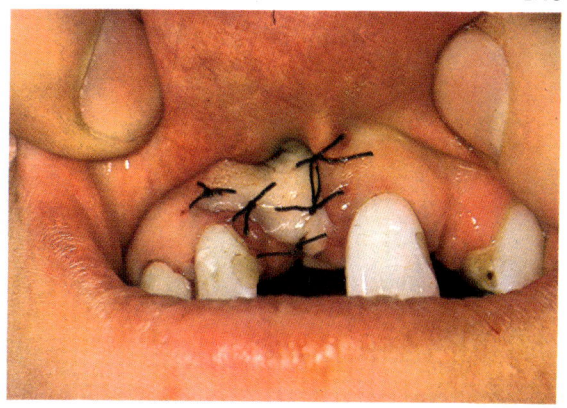

240. The patient shown in **77** and **78** is to be treated by means of a gingival graft, to overcome the aesthetic problem of the discoloured tissue. Subsequently a bridge is to be constructed.

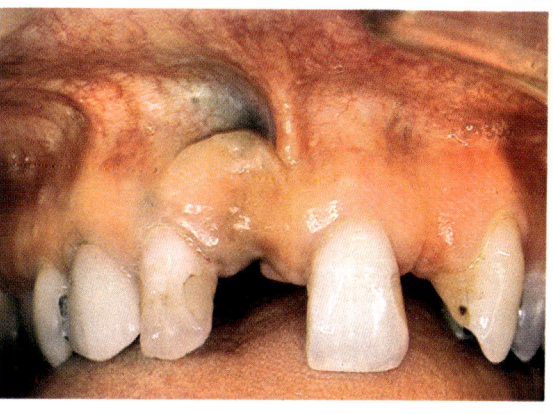

241. A good appearance has been achieved and at eight weeks after surgery the patient is ready for the restorative procedures to be commenced.

The gingival graft procedure may be of value prior to restorative procedures under a variety of circumstances. Where there is minimal width of keratinized gingiva there is the danger that an increase in the concentration of irritants caused by plaque retention at the margins of restorations might result in inflammation and recession. A zone of attached gingiva can be achieved by means of a graft with the aim of establishing a more stable location of the gingival margins.

16. *The laterally repositioned flap*

Introduction

The laterally repositioned flap is used as an alternative to the free gingival graft to treat a localised area of gingival recession. Prior to the procedure it is necessary to diagnose and correct the causative factors. Recession is often associated with a tooth which is prominent in the arch and during treatment this prominence must be corrected by orthodontic means or by removal of tooth tissue by root planing. The patient's toothbrushing technique is assessed and if this is inflicting trauma to the gingiva any necessary modification is made. The shape of any bony dehiscence associated with the recession should be assessed by probing through the soft tissues under local analgesic. There is a better prognosis for the lateral flap procedure when there is a narrow, shallow dehiscence and where there is minimal loss of interproximal bone on either side of the defect. There must be no dehiscence or fenestration of the alveolar plate on the donor tooth, and ideally the gingivae should be relatively thick at the donor site (Douglas 1976).

Operative technique

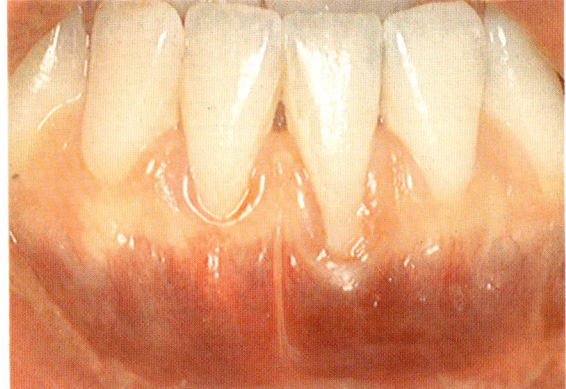

242. This patient is concerned about the recession involving the lower left central incisor. There is an aesthetic problem as she shows the lower anterior gingiva when she speaks. The initial therapy has been completed and a laterally repositioned flap is to be undertaken.

The flap procedure is preferred to a free graft in this case, as there is an insufficient width of gingival tissue on the involved tooth to enable it to be retained and so provide a circumscribed defect suitable for a graft.

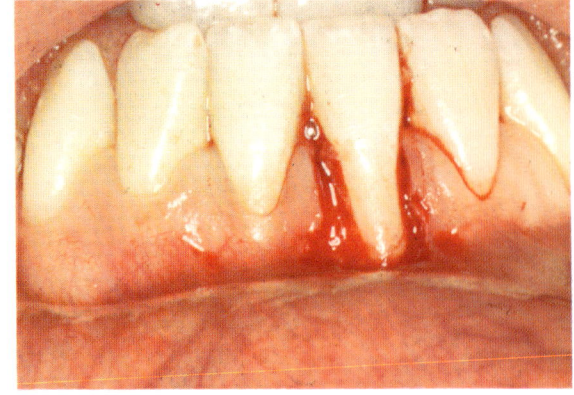

243. The marginal gingiva and sulcular epithelium are removed around the area of recession and the root surface planed. Sufficient tooth tissue is removed to bring the root into alignment with the neighbouring bone margins.

Operative technique

244. A vertical incision is made on the mesial aspect of the lower canine and a flap raised. Sufficient mobility of the tissues must be achieved to enable the flap to be moved to the new site without any tension. Where the gingiva is sufficiently thick a split thickness flap should be used in preference to a full thickness flap; retaining the periosteum reduces alveolar bone resorption during healing and conserves the height of the gingival margin on the donor tooth.

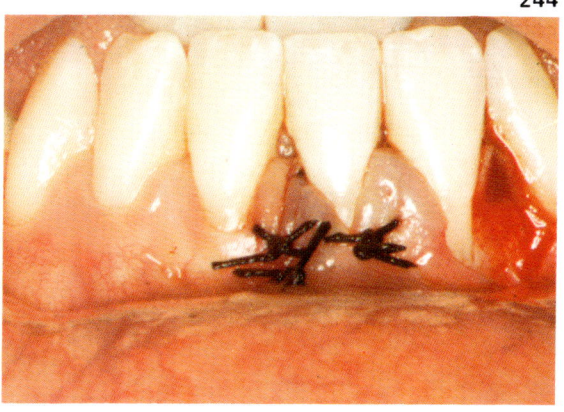

245. The tissues have healed well and the amount of recession has been reduced on the left central incisor, the sulcus on this tooth is 1.5mm deep. There is, however, slightly increased recession on the donor tooth; this is a common sequel to the procedure. Histological studies have shown that the new attachment of the gingiva to the recipient tooth is achieved by cementogenesis and new connective tissue attachment in the apical zone, and by attachment of the junctional epithelium to the tooth more coronally (Sugarman 1969).

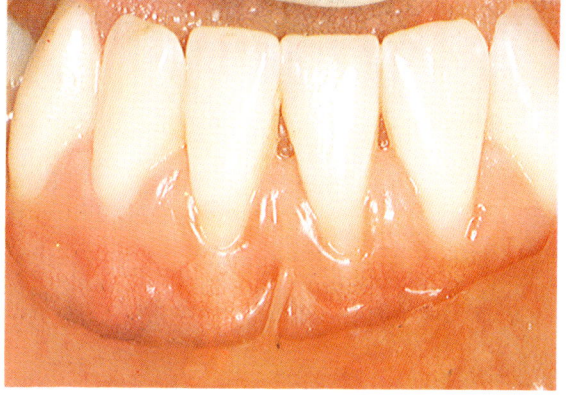

Application of the procedure

246. The recession on this lower right central incisor was associated with a relatively prominent position of the tooth in the arch. The alignment of the tooth in the arch was first improved by orthodontic treatment.

247. Following this a laterally repositioned flap was used to correct the gingival deformity and achieve a zone of keratinized gingival tissue.

Where there is gingival recession on a tooth next to a saddle area the masticatory mucosa of the ridge may be used as a pedicle graft for the laterally repositioned flap procedure.

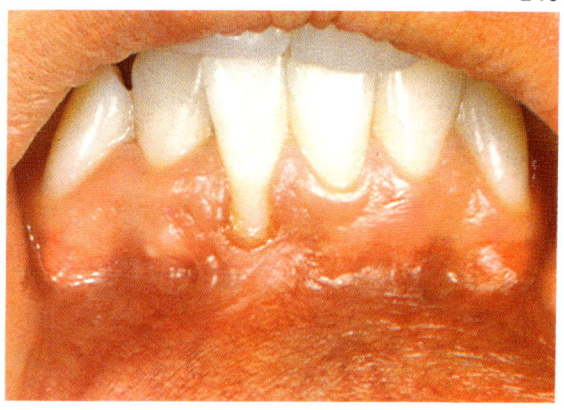

Summary

The procedure is applied mainly to treat localised areas of recession, where there is an aesthetic problem. The success of the procedure depends on the formation of an attachment between the flap and the cementum of the root. Postoperatively there is usually some recurrence of the recession but not to the original level (Smukler 1976). The recently developed coronally repositioned free gingival graft (**238, 239**) is an alternative procedure. Both techniques have a limited application and have an uncertain prognosis.

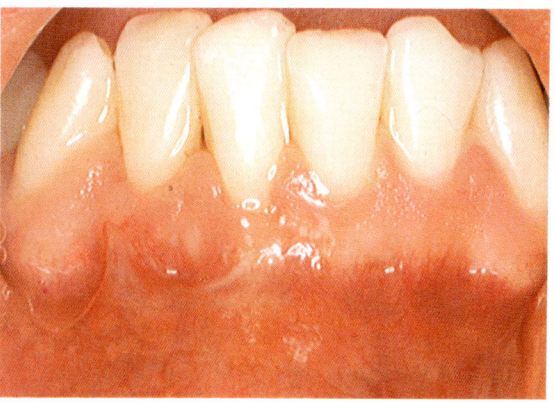

17. Occlusion and periodontal disease

The influence of malocclusion

248. Poulton and Aaronson (1961) demonstrated an association between periodontal disease and increase in incisor overjet and overbite. An increase in overjet predisposes to a lack of lip seal with resultant drying of the anterior gingivae (**39, 40**).

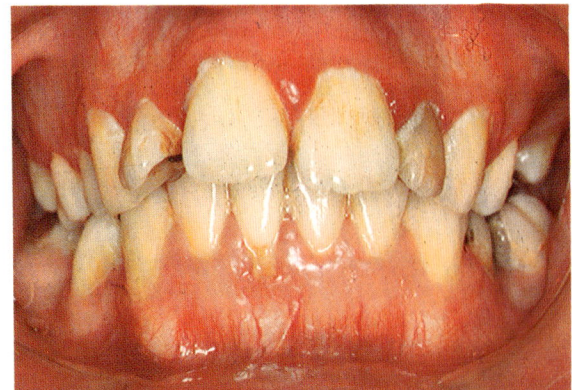

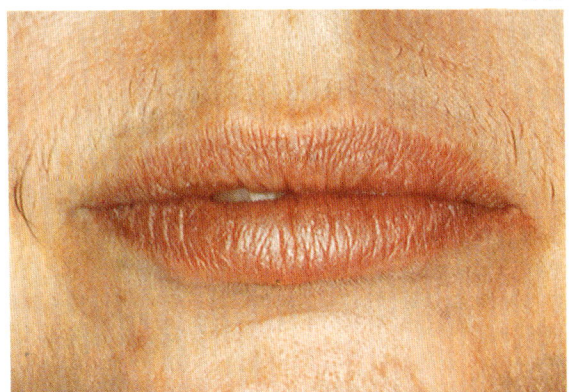

249. Increased overjet may also cause an imbalance of soft tissue forces due to the anterior component of force from the lower lip.

250. On the above patient this anterior force in conjunction with the established periodontitis has resulted in an accelerated rate of bone destruction on the central incisors. The teeth are migrating as a result of these factors.

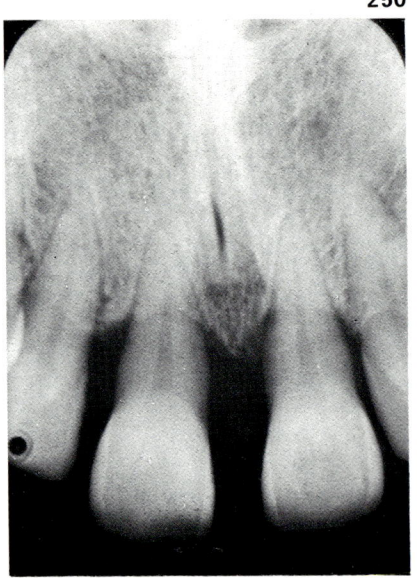

The influence of malocclusion

251. Increased overbite may result in trauma to the palatal gingiva, and food packing around the gingival margins. On this patient palatal abscess formation has resulted and sinuses are discharging through the buccal alveolar bone in the right and left lateral incisor regions. In a patient with Angle Class II division ii malocclusion the lower labial gingiva may also be traumatised by the upper incisor teeth (**13**).

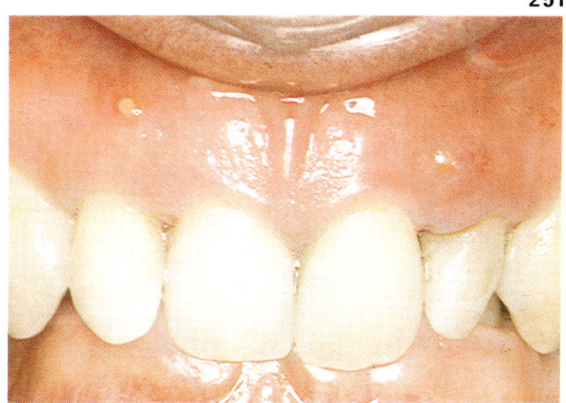

252. A number of studies on adult patients have demonstrated that malaligned teeth predispose to periodontal disease. There have been, however, other studies which have not found this association; the disagreement may be due to differences between the groups of subjects studied. Ainamo (1972) found that, where there was moderately effective plaque control, malaligned teeth had increased plaque deposits and more gingival inflammation, as demonstrated on this patient. In contrast Ainamo found that where oral hygiene was bad both malaligned and regular teeth were uniformly covered with gross plaque deposits, and there was no variation between the teeth in the degree of inflammation.

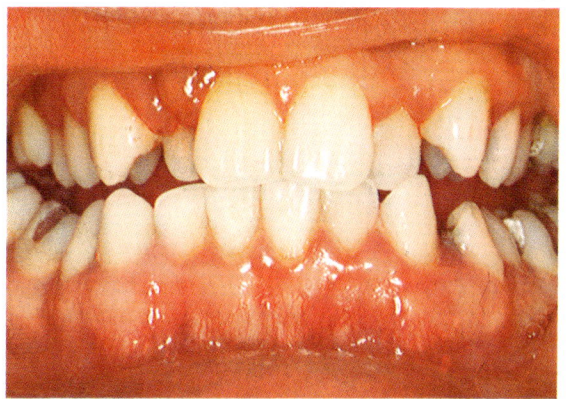

253. Ainamo also observed that patients with very good plaque control were able to remove deposits from malposed teeth, and the gingival condition was therefore uniformly healthy. The patient in **252** has completed a course of periodontal treatment; her oral hygiene is now excellent and the gingival condition is satisfactory. Special oral hygiene equipment may be of value for cleaning imbricated teeth, for example the interspace brush (**115**).

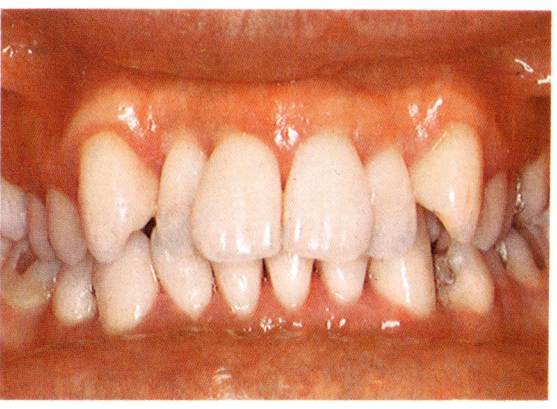

254. Plaque control is of particular importance where cosmetic considerations dictate orthodontic intervention, as an orthodontic appliance tends to increase plaque retention. Zachrisson and co-workers (1972, 1973 and 1974) found that there was a transient increase in gingivitis during orthodontic treatment. Over the treatment period there was also 0.3mm more loss of attachment than for a control group. These findings emphasise the need to provide oral hygiene instruction as part of the orthodontic treatment plan.

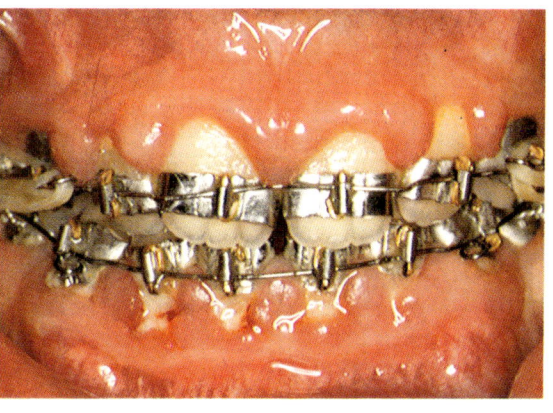

Response of the periodontium to occlusal forces

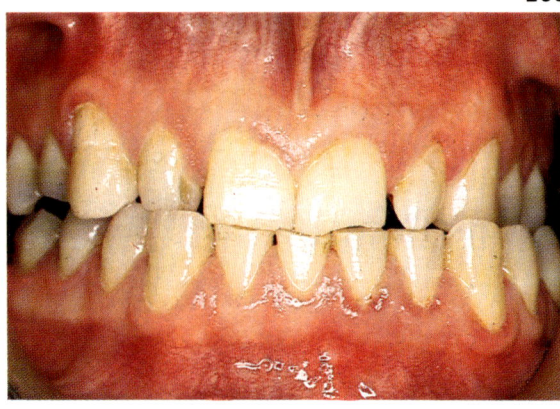

255. The severe attrition on the anterior teeth of this patient has been caused by parafunction. From the degree of attrition it may be deduced that the teeth have been subjected to excessive forces for a prolonged period of time. There is minimal inflammation present and this is confined to the gingival tissues.

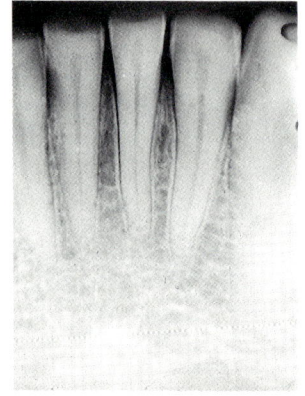

256. In response to these increased occlusal forces there is a thickening of the lamina dura and slight widening of the periodontal ligament space. The response of healthy tissue to excessive force is termed primary trauma, and this can be separated into two phases – a traumatic phase and a post-traumatic phase. During the former there is increased vascularity and resorption of the wall of the socket. In the post-traumatic phase the periodontium has adapted to the occlusal forces with resultant increased mobility, widened periodontal membrane space, reduced density of bone, and reduced crestal height of bone. However the level of attachment remains constant during these changes indicating that when inflammation is confined to the marginal gingiva excessive occlusal forces do not accelerate the progression of periodontal disease (Svanberg 1974, Polson *et al* 1976).

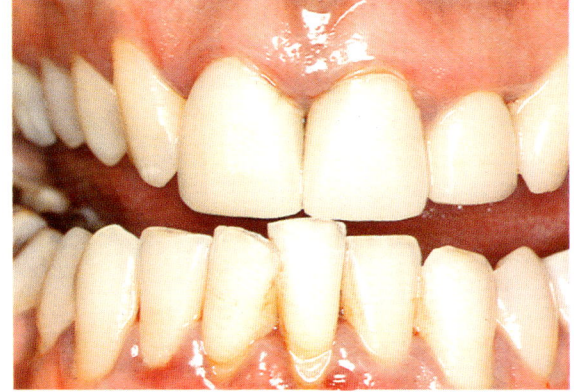

257. For this patient most of the occlusal force in protrusion is taken by the lower central incisor. This tooth is periodontally involved.

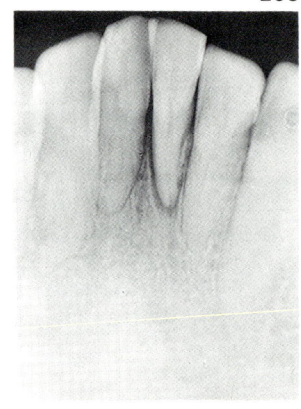

258. The radiograph shows that there is widening of the periodontal membrane space, caused by the response of the tissues to the excessive occlusal loads. In contrast to the first patient the inflammation has progressed to involve the supporting structures. When a tooth is affected by periodontitis and is also involved with occlusal trauma the rate of progression of the periodontal destruction is increased by the vascular changes in the periodontal membrane and by the alterations of the alveolar bone morphology brought about by excessive occlusal forces (Svanberg and Lindhe 1973, and Lindhe and Svanberg 1974). See also **269** and **270**.

Response of the periodontium to occlusal forces

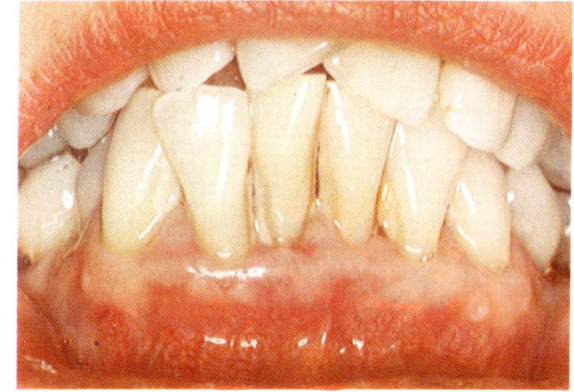

259. Advanced periodontal disease has resulted in the loss of over half the bony investment of these teeth. The reduction in periodontal support has resulted in normal occlusal forces now becoming traumatogenic, thereby causing changes in the periodontal membrane, termed secondary trauma.

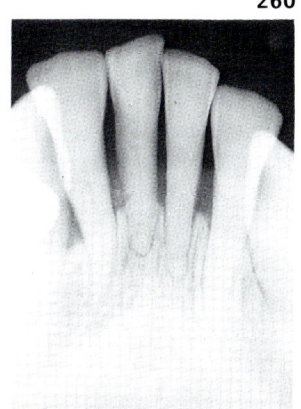

260. The radiographs of the above patient show advanced bone loss. Involvement of the periodontium with secondary trauma is accelerating the rate of periodontal destruction.

In summary, recent research has shown that for the healthy periodontium or where there is inflammation confined to the gingiva excessive occlusal forces do not cause loss of periodontal attachment. Where there is periodontitis however the rate of periodontal destruction is increased by traumatogenic occlusal forces, as a result of the vascular, morphological and cellular changes in the periodontium brought about by the excessive forces.

The migration of teeth

261. The aetiology of migration of teeth is often complex. The underlying cause of the movement is usually a net anterior force acting on teeth with reduced periodontal support. The force may be caused by various factors: (a) habits, (b) forces exerted by the soft tissues, (c) occlusal factors.

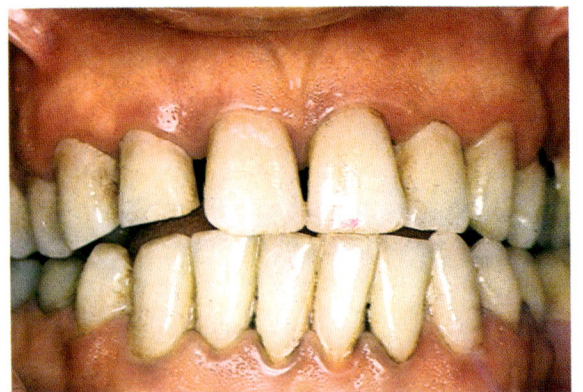

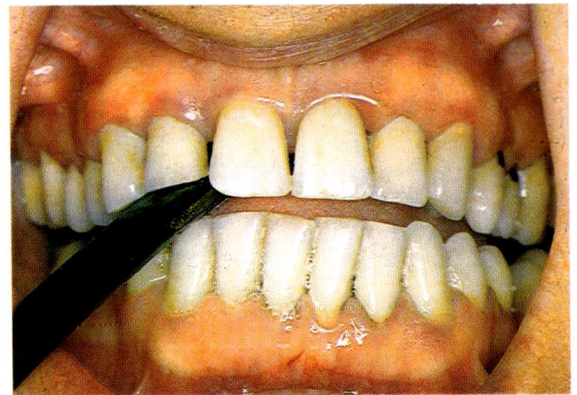

262. In the case of the above patient the force causing the movement of the periodontally involved anterior teeth was found to be his habit of pipe smoking. Sometimes habits may be difficult to detect; these may include finger or nail biting, pressing pencils or other objects against the teeth and chewing or sucking the lips, tongue or cheek.

263. The radiograph shows increased bone loss on the affected tooth caused by combined periodontal destruction and trauma from occlusion.

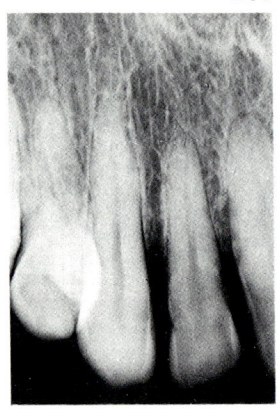

264. This patient complains that a space has developed between her central incisors and she has noticed that she tends to put her tongue into this space. At rest the lower lip lies on the incisal edge of the upper incisors or sometimes behind them.

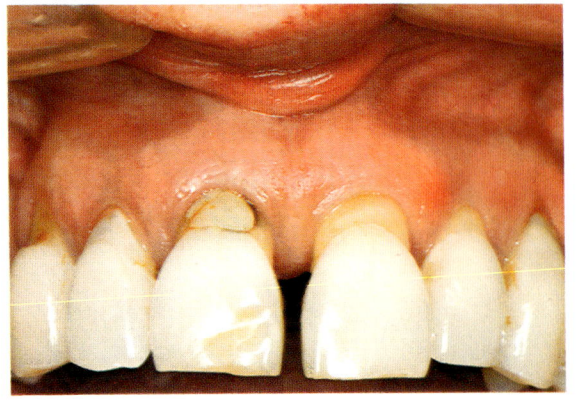

The migration of teeth

265. There is generalised periodontal pocketing and this is deeper on the palatal aspect where probing reveals a depth of 6mm.

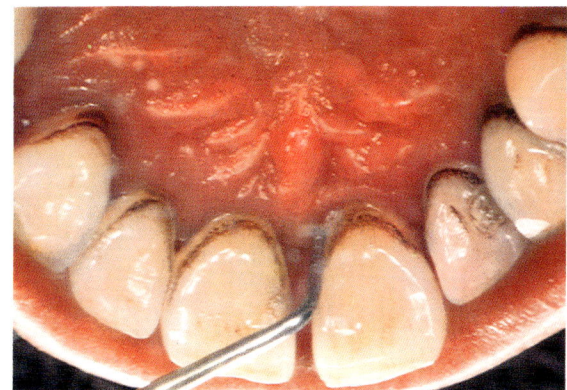

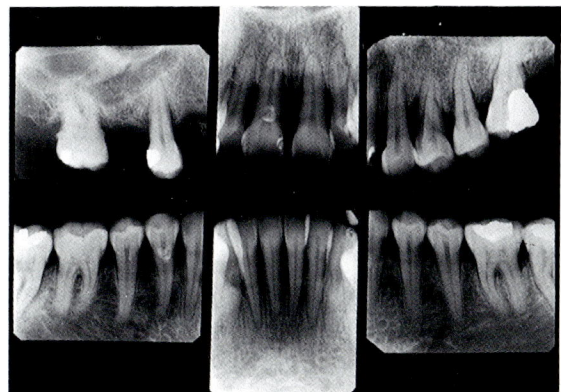

266. The radiographs show generalised bone loss due to periodontal disease; this is severe around the upper anterior teeth. There are angular osseous defects around the upper right second premolar and some of the other teeth. The configuration of the bone and the enhanced rate of destruction on these teeth is suggestive of trauma from occlusion.

267. Analysis of the occlusion of this patient reveals that there is minimal incisor overjet. There are interferences in the retruded contact position caused by bilateral premature contacts.

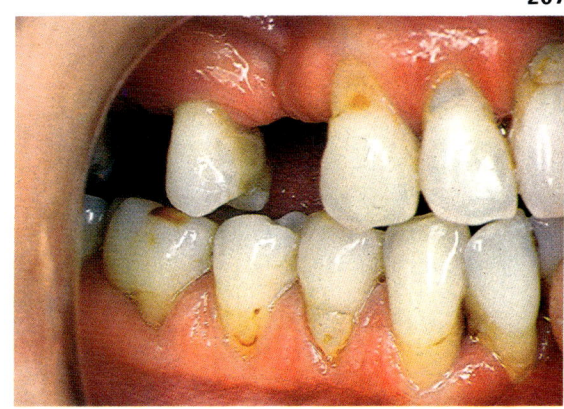

268. There is a 3mm anterior displacement into the intercuspal position. This can be seen by comparing the relationship between the distal aspect of the upper right canine and the lower first premolar in **267** and **268**. The displacement results in an anterior force being applied to the upper incisor teeth which is a contributory cause of the migration (Wise 1977). The complete treatment plan must involve plaque control and scaling, occlusal adjustment, orthodontic treatment, periodontal surgery and prosthetic reconstruction (see Appendix 4).

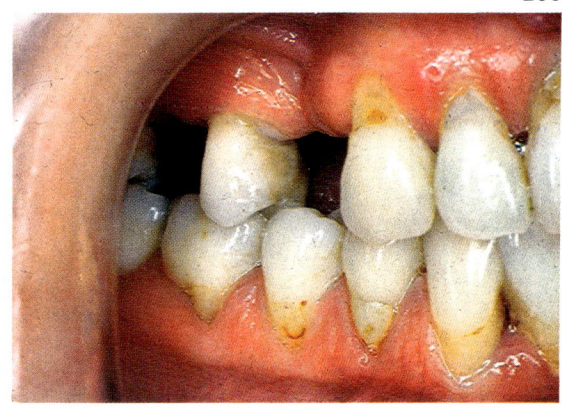

18. Occlusal adjustment

Introduction

According to Sugarman (1970) prophylactic occlusal adjustment is contraindicated. He defines the clinical criteria for adjustment as being:

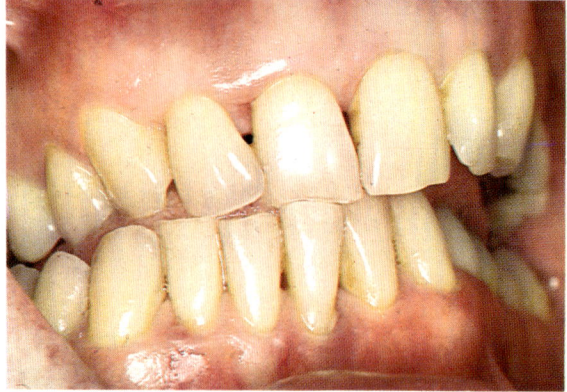

269. Where there is increased mobility clinically, or where there is uneven distribution of forces resulting in secondary trauma.

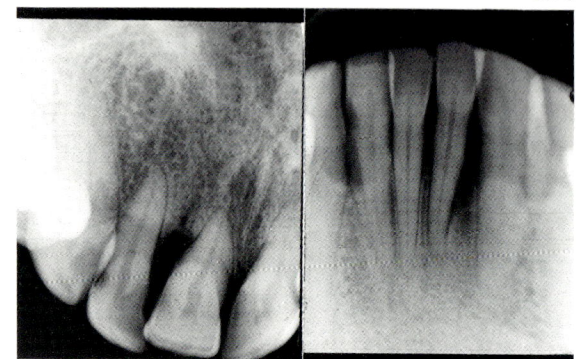

270. Where there is a widened periodontal ligament space on the radiographs or where bone loss is advanced, with the danger of secondary trauma.

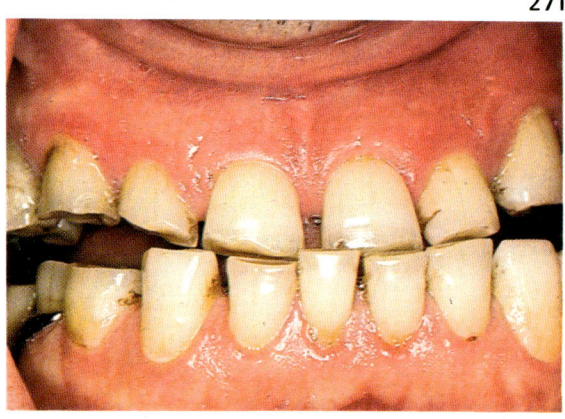

271. Where there is bruxism indicated here by the degree of attrition, or where there is pain caused by dysfunction.

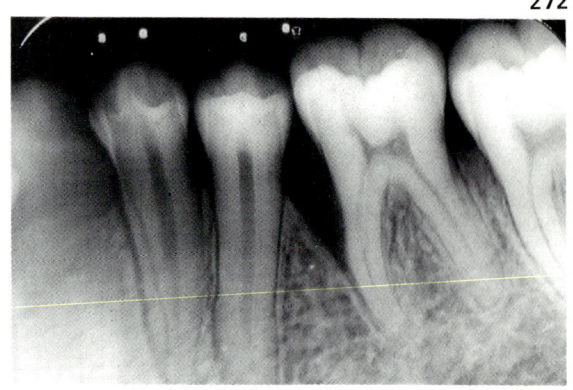

272. Glickman & Smulow (1969) state that infrabony pockets and angular osseous defects are not pathognomic of trauma from occlusion; however their presence is suggestive of traumatogenic factors and when they are present the occlusion of the patient should be assessed.

Retruded and intercuspal positions

273. Simple occlusal analysis can be carried out directly in the mouth. Occlusal contacts in the retruded axis should first be assessed. A posterior force is applied to the patient's chin and the mandible is moved up and down by the operator. The patient is encouraged to relax the jaw muscles.

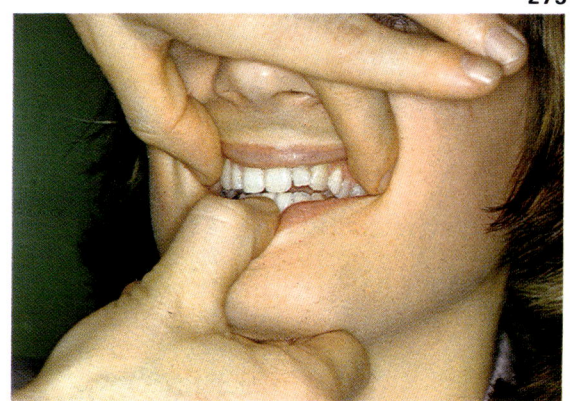

274. The point of first contact is observed, in this case the first contact is in the premolar region. Any deviation or interference in the articulation from this position to that of full intercuspation is noted. Premature contacts are often caused by malposed teeth, as here, or incorrectly contoured restorations.

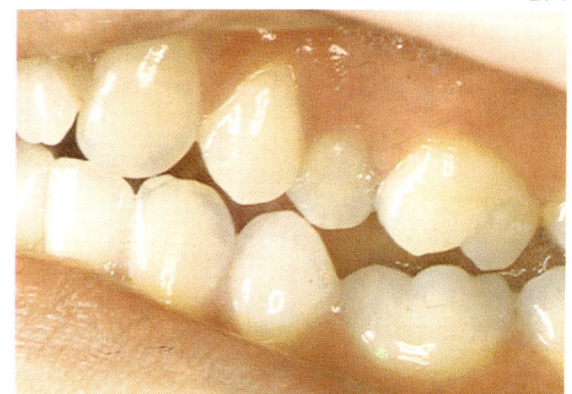

275. This patient was complaining of pain in the right temporo-mandibular joint. Geering (1974) noted a correlation between pain or functional disturbance of the masticatory system, and occlusal interferences on the same side of the mouth. Removal of the interference on the above patient was followed by relief of her symptoms.

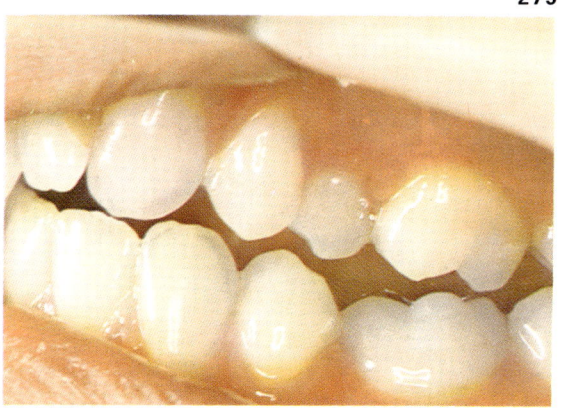

276. The correction of interferences in the retruded axis may involve a choice between the deepening of a fossa or the reduction of a cusp. In the upper diagram the lower buccal cusp is in premature contact on intercuspation but is in the correct relationship on both working and non-working excursions. The cusp should therefore not be adjusted, rather the fossa should be deepened on the upper tooth. In the lower diagram the lower buccal cusp is high in the intercuspal position and on both lateral excursions, and this cusp is therefore adjusted rather than the upper fossa.

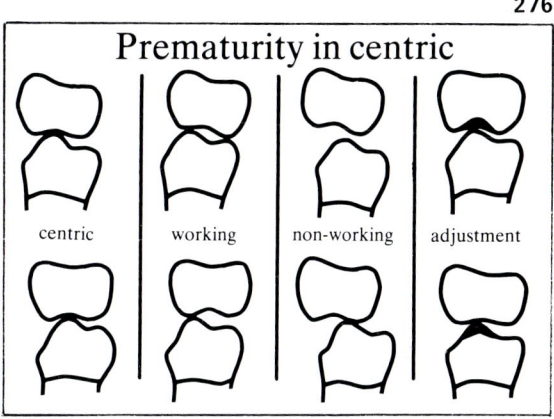

Lateral excursions

277. The occlusion is then checked in lateral excursion on the working side. The most common occlusion on the working side in the natural dentition is the 'canine guided'. As the mandible moves into lateral excursion on the working side the articulation is guided by the canine, which causes the premolar and molar teeth to come out of occlusion.

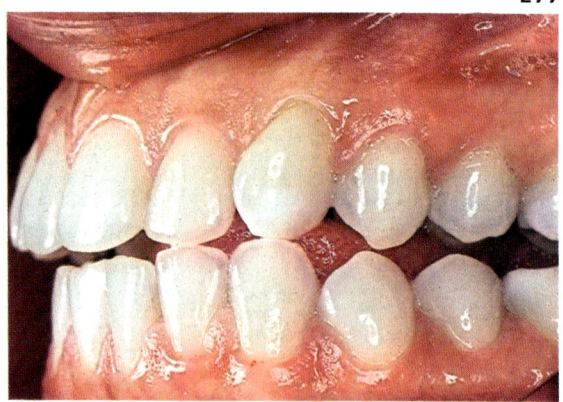

278. Where there is periodontitis a canine guided occlusion may result in excessive force being applied to the guiding teeth with a resultant enhanced rate of breakdown.

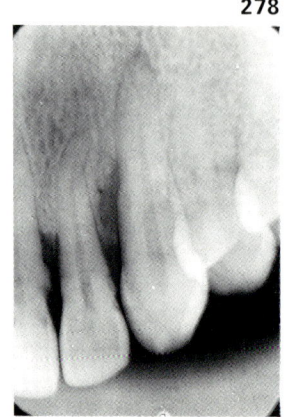

279. The less common type of occlusion of the working side is 'group function'. In lateral excursion all the buccal teeth are in contact on the working side. In this patient the occlusal relationship appears to have resulted from attrition of the upper canine tooth.

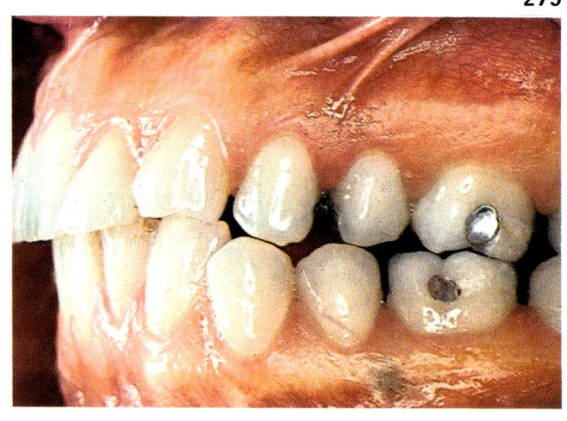

280. It is frequently beneficial to create group function in lateral excursion for periodontally involved teeth. This enables the load on the working side to be distributed according to the relative quality and quantity of support of the individual teeth. The articulation of the cusps is adjusted by selectively grinding the buccal upper cusps or the lingual lower cusps, i.e. the cusps which are not in contact in the position of intercuspation.

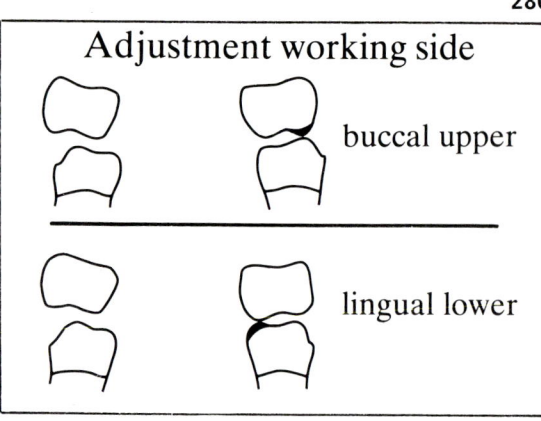

Lateral excursions

281. This patient has gross attrition on the posterior teeth due to bruxism. There is controversy about the treatment of parafunction. The provision of a bite guard with a flat occlusal surface for wear at night (see **290**) may reduce bruxism in some patients, and will decrease the lateral forces applied to the teeth by preventing intercuspation.

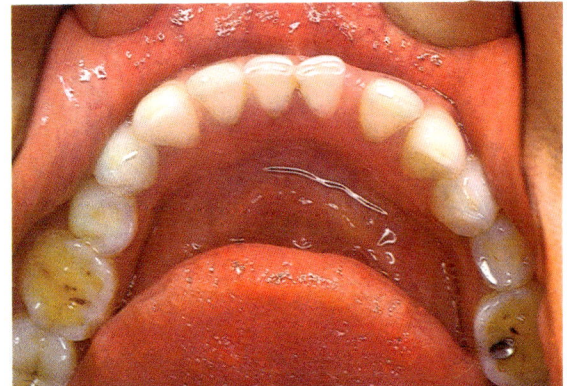

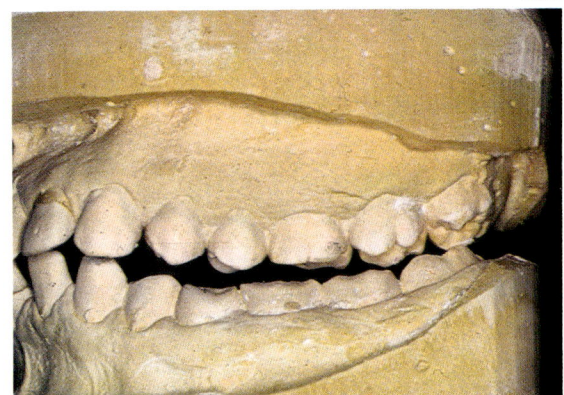

282. It has been suggested that premature contacts predispose to parafunction (Glickman 1972). On the above patient there is a premature contact on the non-working side.

283. The removal of this premature contact should be designed so that contacts in the intercuspal position and working excursions are maintained. By adjusting the inclines on the involved teeth the change in actual cusp height is minimised.

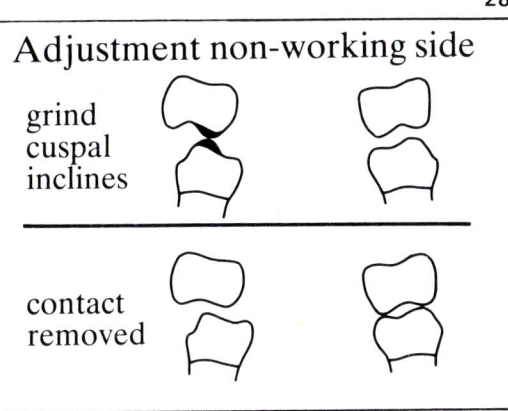

Protrusive excursion

284. For the patient with periodontal disease the most common adjustment in protrusion is the redistribution of occlusal load between the anterior teeth. In the natural dentition there is usually no contact of the molar teeth in protrusive excursion.

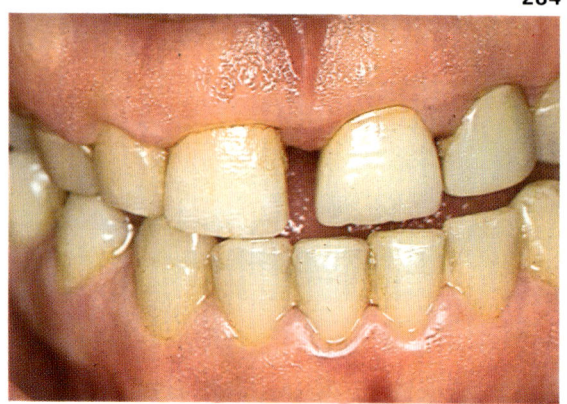

285. Adjustment was indicated on this patient because the tooth in premature contact in protrusion had jeopardised support, and was therefore subject to secondary trauma.

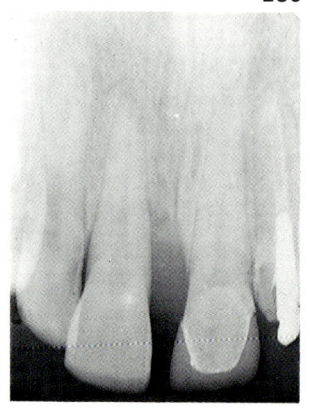

286. Green indicator wax may be used to detect premature contacts.

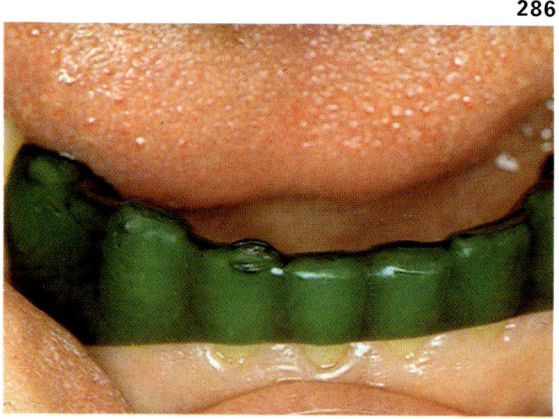

287. Alternatively, thin articulating paper may be used. The inclination of the incisal edges of the upper teeth should be adjusted rather than the lower; the incisal edges of the lower teeth should be preserved to maintain contact in the intercuspal position. Failure to observe this may result in over-eruption of the lower incisors.

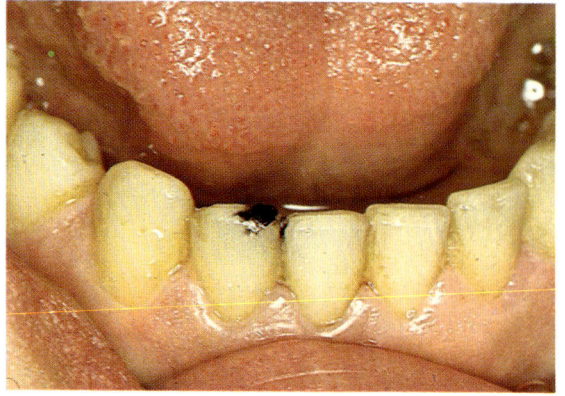

Protrusive excursion

288. The analysis of more complex occlusal problems may necessitate the taking of a face bow registration, so that the models may be mounted in an articulator.

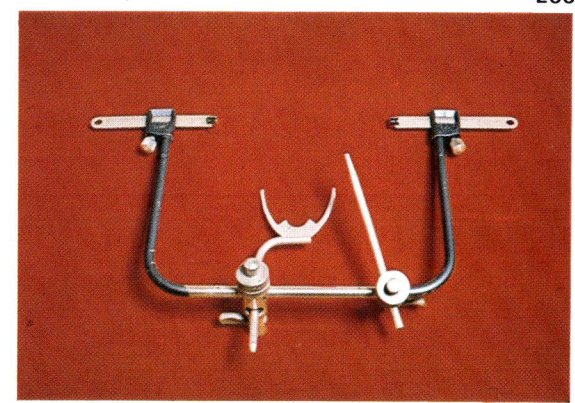

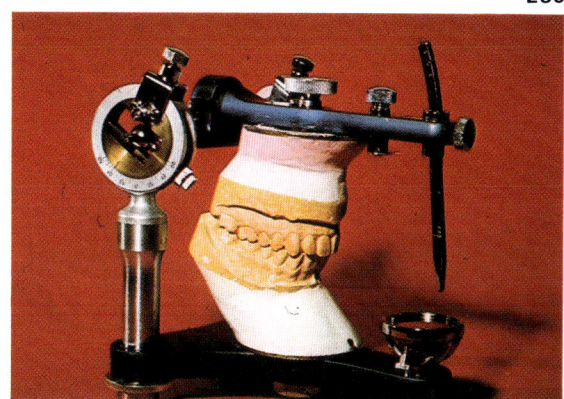

289. Analysis and provisional occlusal adjustment may then be carried out on the models with improved access and visibility. There is a wide variety of articulators available, this is the Dentatus model. Gnathological articulators are more accurate but are very complicated and time consuming to use.

19. The rôle of splints in periodontal therapy

Introduction

The rôle of splints in the treatment of periodontal disease includes:
(1) The temporary stabilisation of teeth with advanced bone loss during operative procedures.
(2) The distribution of occlusal forces where after periodontal therapy there is still secondary trauma indicated by increasing mobility.
(3) Retention after orthodontic tooth movement.
(4) Distribution of forces exerted by a prosthesis on the abutment teeth (see **326**).

Temporary splints

Temporary splints are used during the treatment of teeth with severely reduced support where there is the possibility that the teeth might be subluxed or extracted inadvertently during the scaling or surgical procedures. In the initial healing phase after periodontal surgery there is a temporary increase in mobility caused by the inflammatory response to surgical trauma. Where the teeth being treated have advanced bone loss this transient reduction in the quality of periodontal support may be sufficient to result in the induction of secondary trauma. If the adaptive potential of the periodontal ligament is exceeded the mobility will continue to increase. Temporary splinting should be used prior to surgical treatment on teeth with severely reduced support to prevent this secondary trauma.

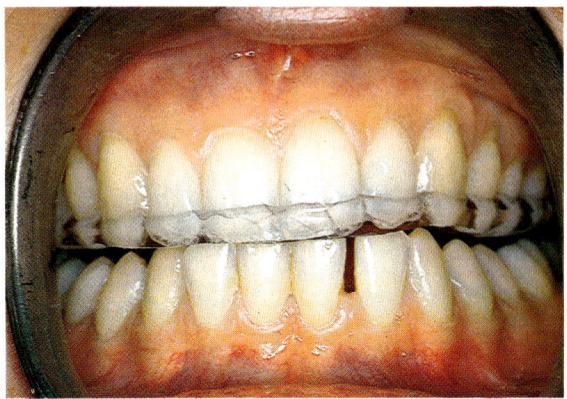

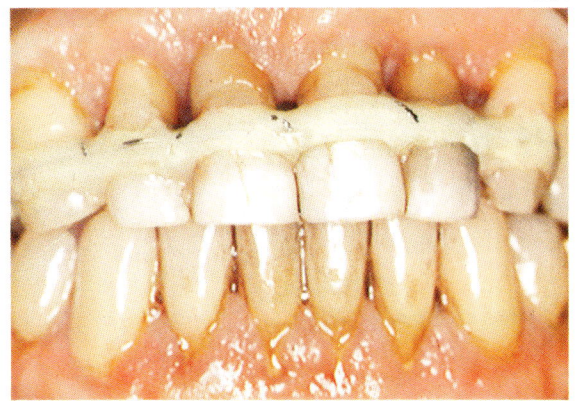

290. One of the simplest forms of temporary splint is the bite guard. When used as a splint the appliance should be designed so that it covers the incisal edges and occlusal surfaces of all the teeth in the arch to prevent over-eruption. It is bulky and should therefore only be used for relatively short periods of stabilisation or for wear at night only.

291. The wire and acrylic splint may also be used for temporary stabilisation (Clark *et al* 1969). The appliance must be kept well clear of the gingival margins and interproximal spaces to permit cleaning. This type of splint is not suitable for long periods of use, as it is liable to fracture and to marginal leakage with resultant caries (see **204**). The appearance of this type of splint is poor.

Semi-permanent splints

Semi-permanent splints are indicated when splinting is required for longer periods of time. They enable the stability of the occlusion after treatment to be assessed prior to considering the need to provide a permanent splint. There are disadvantages, for example some form of tooth preparation is usually required although sometimes existing restorations can be used to prevent having to cut sound tooth tissue. Another disadvantage is that materials employed generally have a low shear strength, and as there are heavy stresses between the splinted teeth fractures of these splints are quite common.

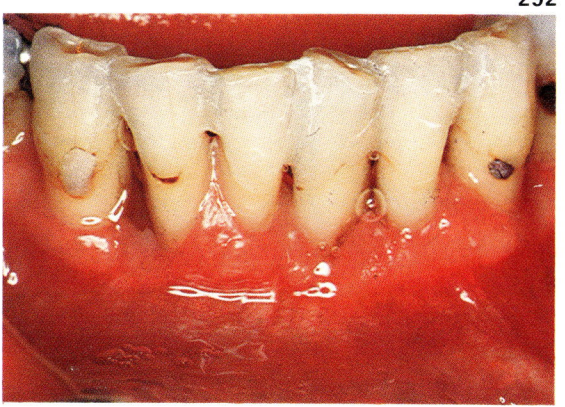

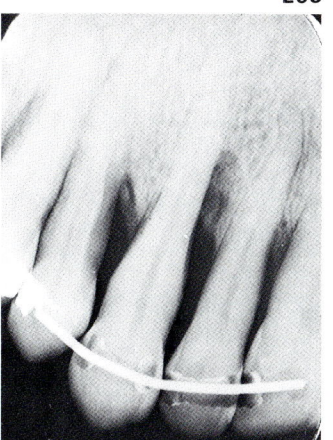

292. A composite restorative material may be used on etched enamel to join the interproximal surfaces of adjoining teeth.

An alternative technique is to cut interproximal cavities in the teeth to be splinted; the teeth are linked with staple shaped pins cemented into holes cut in dentine. After lining the cavities, the teeth are restored with resin or composite restorations.

293. The upper anterior teeth on this patient have been stabilised by means of a stainless steel wire which is cemented with resin into a continuous palatal groove cut in the teeth. The same principle may be used for posterior teeth, the groove being cut in the occlusal surface or in existing amalgam restorations (Cianco and Nisengard 1975).

Removable splints

This type of splint offers the advantage that it can easily be removed so that the mobility of the teeth can be reassessed. The appliance may be left off for a period to enable the longer term stability to be determined.

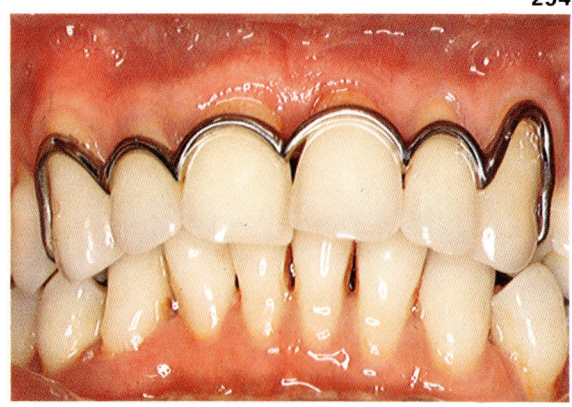

294. The periodontal treatment for this patient has included plaque control, occlusal adjustment and periodontal surgery. His complaint was that he found the upper anterior teeth were too loose to enable him to incise with them. The provision of this chrome cobalt splint with a continuous clasp has restored function to these teeth. Aesthetically it is acceptable to this patient as he has a low lip line when he speaks or smiles.

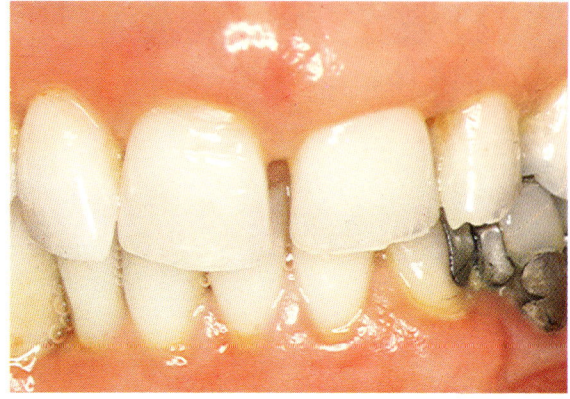

295. This patient has a chronic periodontitis and the resultant bone loss has been contributory to the migration of the incisor teeth. Other factors which caused this movement were an anterior slide into the intercuspal relationship and soft tissue forces.

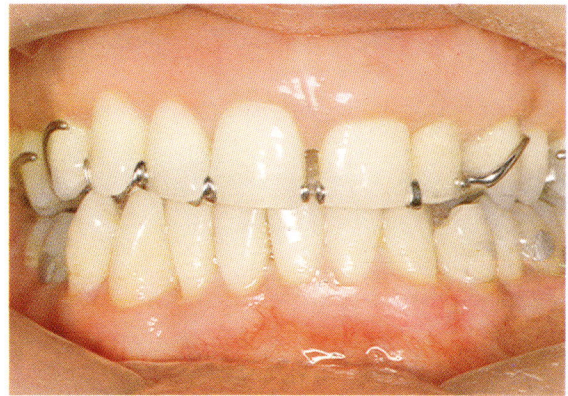

296. The periodontal treatment for the above patient has been completed; this has included correction of the occlusion. A chrome cobalt splint has been fitted to stabilise the teeth.

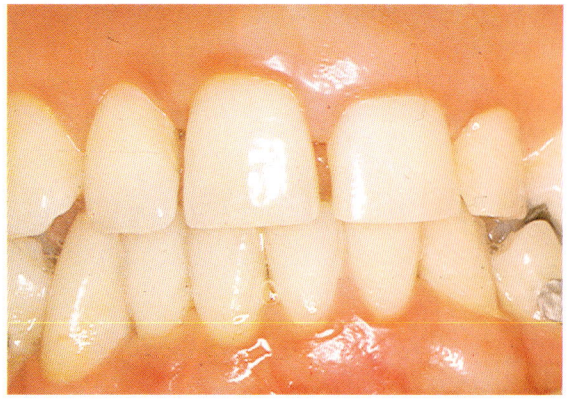

297. After a period of wearing the retainer the upper front teeth have been found to be stable. The appliance is no longer worn and continuing reassessment over a ten year period has revealed that there has been no migration or increase in mobility, in spite of plaque control being only moderately effective.

Removable splints

298. The Von Weisenfluh system is another type of removable splint. Parallel pin holes are drilled in the cingulum regions of the teeth to be splinted. Stainless steel thimbles are then cemented into the holes and an impression taken.

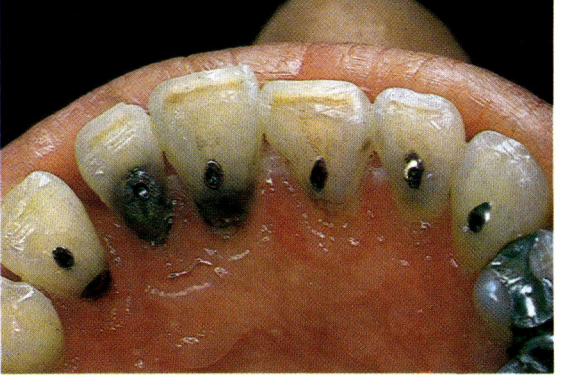

299. The chrome cobalt framework is retained by clasps and has pins which fit into the thimbles. The disadvantages of this system are that it requires the cutting of sound tooth tissue, and that even minor movement of one of the teeth will result in the corresponding pin losing alignment with its thimble, and the splint will then not fit.

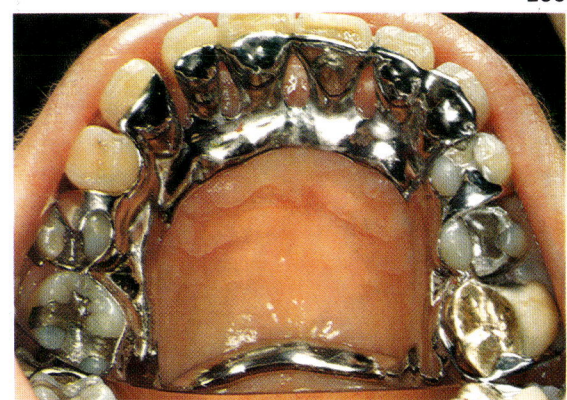

Endodontic implant

300. Stabilisation of a single tooth may be achieved without involving the neighbouring teeth by means of the endodontic implant. This consists of a metal post which is extended through the apex into the periapical bone (Frank 1967).

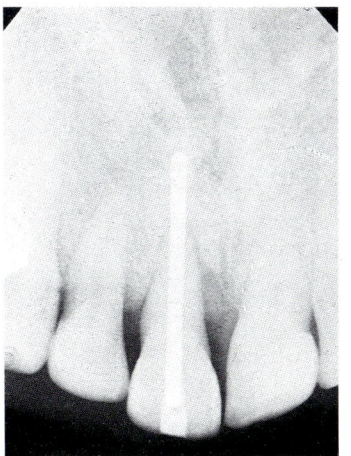

Permanent splints

A variety of intracoronal and extracoronal retainers have been used for splinting teeth. It is necessary that the restorations are sufficiently rigid to resist torsional forces or the cement seal will be broken. The types of preparation which may be used include MOD inlays with cuspal cover, three-quarter crowns, or pin-ledge preparations. Hard gold must be used if there is to be sufficient retention and resistance to torsion.

301. This patient has been fitted with a non-parallel pin splint. It consists of a gold casting on the lingual surfaces of the lower anterior teeth.

302. This is cemented into position and retained by screws which are inserted into holes drilled through each of the teeth to be splinted and then screwed into the lingual casting. The screw heads can be countersunk and restored with silicate or resin (Weissman 1965).

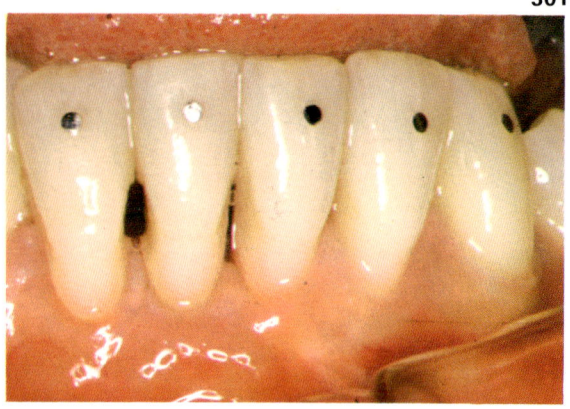

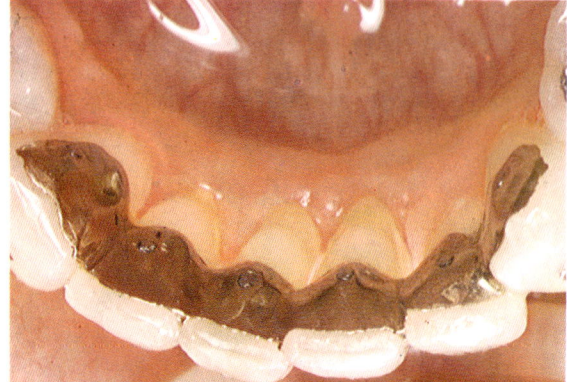

303. The best retention is provided by full crown restorations, but these should only be used in preference to partial cover when there are other indications for them, for example where the teeth are heavily restored. This patient shows that an excellent aesthetic result may be achieved, in spite of considerable recession of the gingival margins caused by periodontal surgery. The edges of the crowns have been kept supragingivally and these have been well tolerated by the tissues.

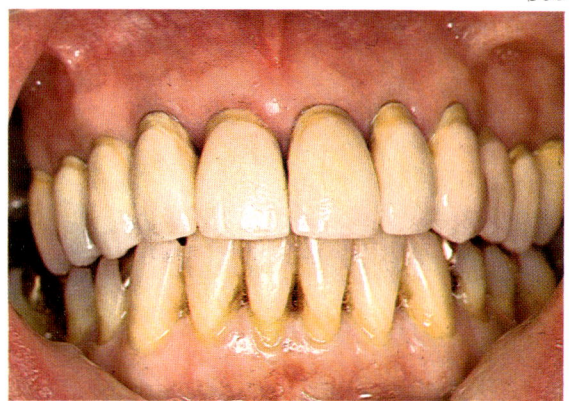

20. Periodontics and restorative dentistry

Conservative dentistry

At the microscopic level it is impossible to achieve perfect marginal adaptation between a restoration and tooth tissue. The degree of marginal discrepancy depends on the material used and on the operative technique. The defect which results offers a retentive site which is shielded from both mechanical and physiological cleansing agents, and rapid colonisation by bacteria ensues. The metabolites produced by these microorganisms have minimal effect on the soft tissues when the margins of the restorations are placed supragingivally. However when they are placed level with the crest of the gingiva or subgingivally their aetiological potential is progressively increased. Examples of periodontal disease associated with defective margins have already been shown (see 36 and 37).

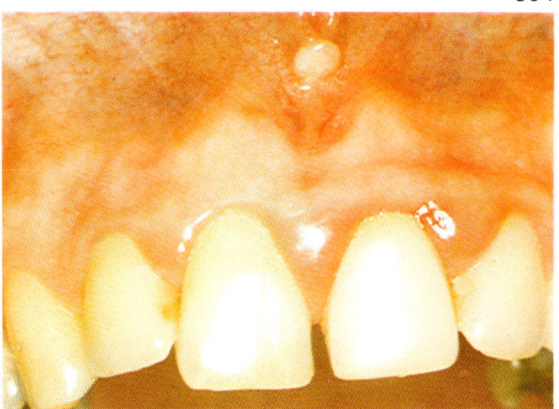

304. The jacket crown on the left central incisor was fitted four years previously; the margins were placed subgingivally for aesthetic reasons. Probing reveals defective margins on all aspects of the tooth. The patient's oral hygiene is poor and consequently there is an early generalised periodontitis. Around the crowned tooth the exacerbated plaque retention has resulted in more severe inflammation.

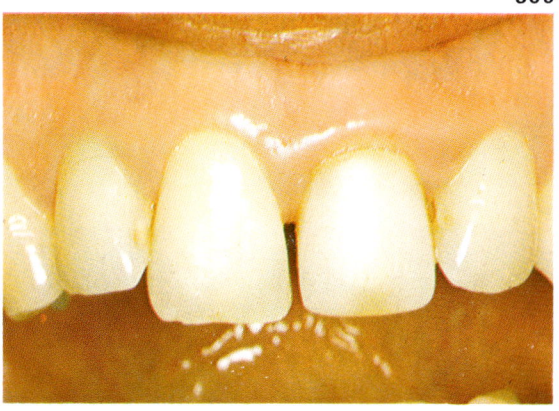

305. It is essential for periodontal disease to be treated before advanced restorative procedures are undertaken. Plaque control and removal of deposits have resulted in reduction of oedema and consquent improvement in tissue contour.

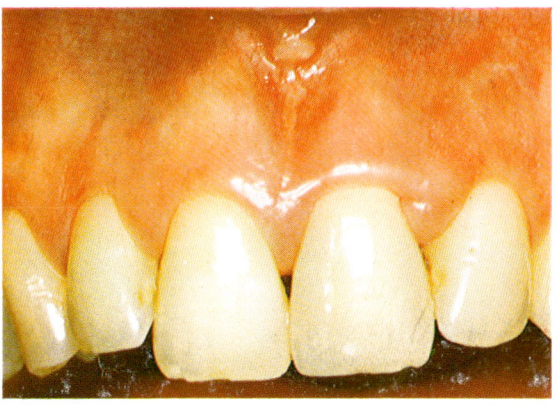

306. Following localised gingivectomy a porcelain jacket crown with good marginal adaptation has been placed. For aesthetic reasons it was necessary to place the labial margin subgingivally. The anatomical sulcus is only 0.5mm deep and the subgingival extension of the margin should not exceed this. On the other surfaces of the tooth the margins were kept above the gingiva. There is a recurrent gingivitis associated with the subgingival margins in spite of good marginal fit.

Prosthetic dentistry

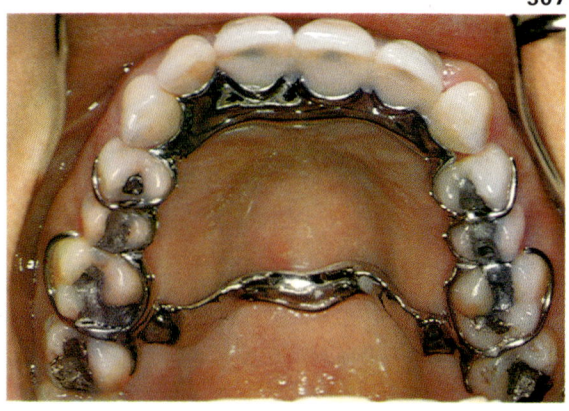

307. The wearing of a dental prosthesis inevitably increases plaque retention. This effect can be minimised by giving the patient oral hygiene instruction with particular emphasis being placed on cleaning the area covered by the prosthesis. A tooth-borne design of prosthesis as illustrated with minimal gingival cover is well tolerated by the periodontal tissues. In the case of free end saddle prostheses, dentures should be designed to use combined tooth and tissue support.

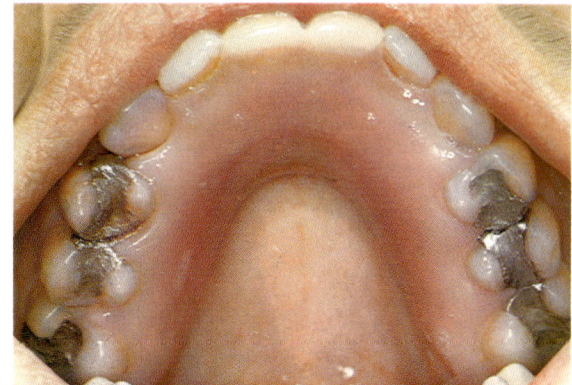

308. This acrylic tissue-borne denture has many design faults: there are no clasps or occlusal rests and there is excessive coverage of the gingival margins. The prosthesis has been worn for six years without being relined.

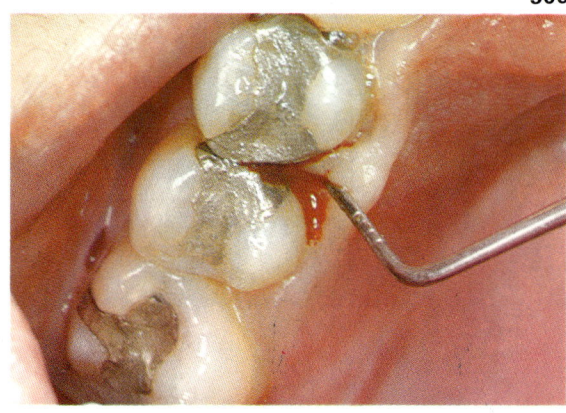

309. Enhanced plaque retention at the gingival margins has resulted in gingival hyperplasia and periodontitis.

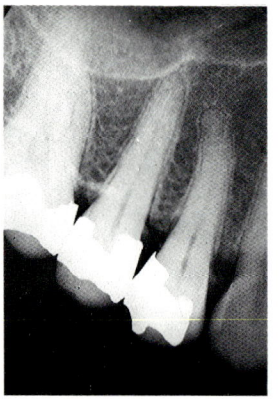

310. The degree of alveolar bone loss can be seen on the radiographs.

Prosthetic dentistry

311. Oral hygiene instruction, scaling and periodontal surgery have been carried out. The pockets have been eliminated and there is a satisfactory gingival contour; the upper arch is now ready for a replacement prosthesis.

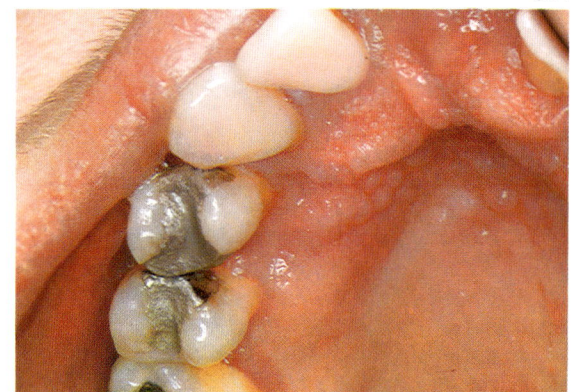

312. A prosthesis may be used to improve the aesthetics after periodontal surgery. This patient had new jacket crowns placed shortly before being referred for periodontal therapy. The advanced restorative procedures should have been postponed until the completion of all surgical treatment, so that the crown margins could be placed in the desired position relative to the definitive gingival level (see **303** and Appendix 4).

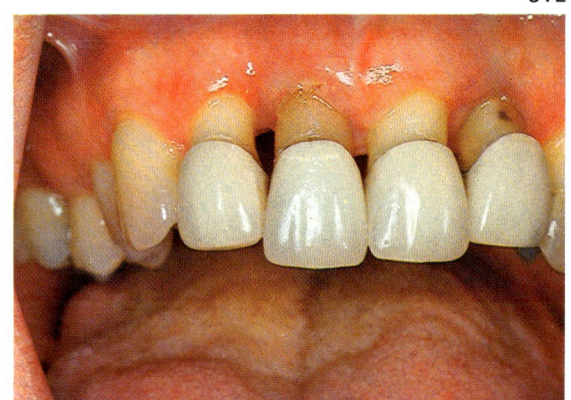

313. The patient has achieved excellent plaque control and because of this it was decided that the provision of an acrylic veneer would not be detrimental to the health of the tissues. The impression for the construction of a veneer is taken in a laboratory made tray, which is designed to enable a labial path of withdrawal to be used. The acrylic of the veneer is extended interdentally to provide retention. The patient leaves the prosthesis out at night and for part of the day depending on her social activities.

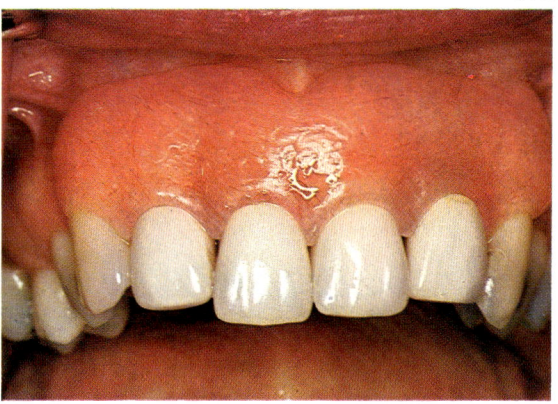

Endodontic therapy

The importance of differentiating between a periodontal and periapical abscess has been mentioned (**92, 93**). Where there is combined pathology it is important to establish the primary cause, as this will influence the treatment. For example, where there is a periapical abscess discharging through the periodontal ligament, endodontic therapy will usually result in spontaneous repair of the fistula. In contrast, where a periodontal defect appears to be closely associated with the apex of a tooth but the pulp is still vital, periodontal therapy is indicated without resource to endodontic therapy.

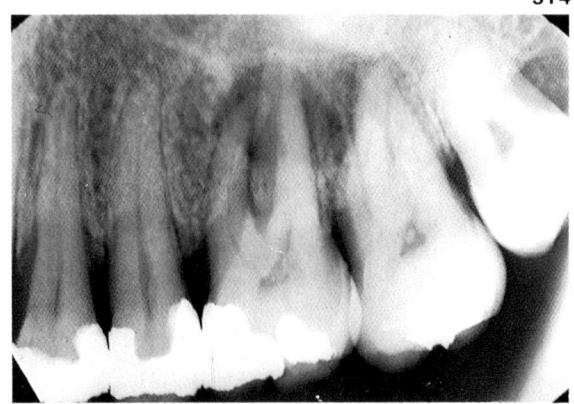

314. There is a periapical abscess on the first molar, which is discharging through the periodontal membrane into the gingival sulcus. The primary cause of the pathology is the non-vital pulp.

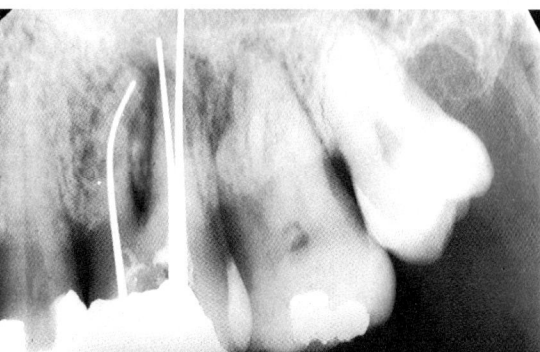

315. Endodontic treatment has just been completed. On the radiograph the apical lesion is still present, and one can also see that there is furcation involvement possibly due to an accessary canal.

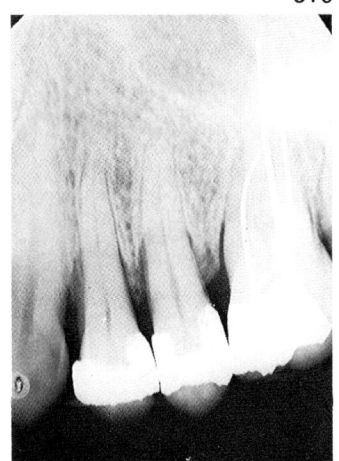

316. Six months later the bone rarefaction has resolved without further treatment. The furcation could no longer be probed.

Endodontic therapy

317. It is less common to find coexistent periodontal and periapical pathology. In this patient the maxillary left lateral incisor is involved with dual pathology. There is a buccal sinus draining from a periapical lesion and a probe is being used to demonstrate the presence of periodontal pocketing. Periodontal and endodontic therapy are to be combined.

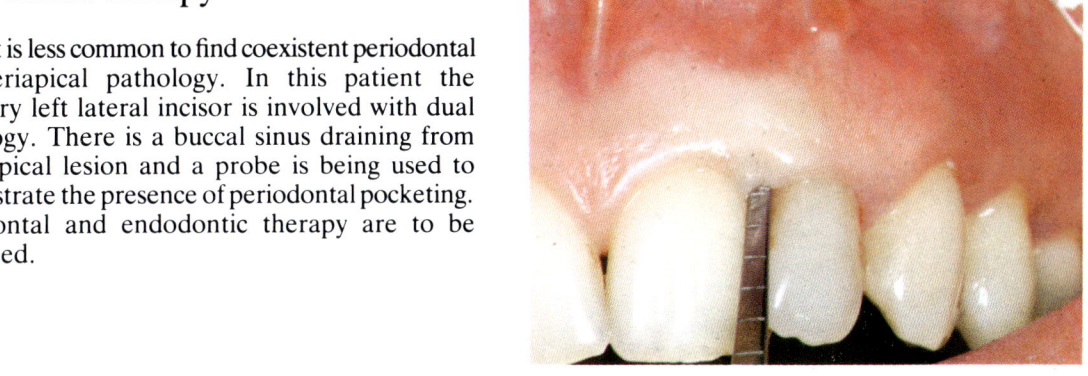

318. Following the plaque control phase of therapy the inverse bevel flap procedure is being used to eliminate the periodontal pockets.

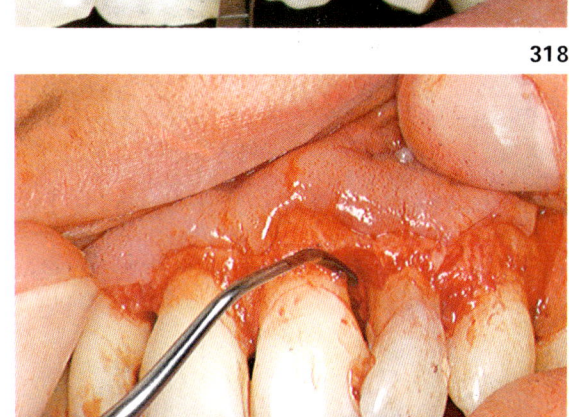

319. The flap reflection is increased to gain access to the apical region. Following curettage of inflammatory tissue from the periapical defect, the apex is trimmed and a small cavity is prepared. A retrograde root filling is then placed.

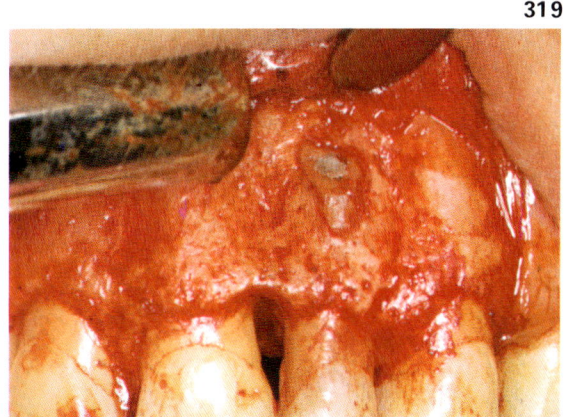

320. At the reassessment four weeks after surgery it is found that the pockets have been eliminated and the sinus has resolved.

The application of endodontic therapy in the treatment of furcation defects by amputation of roots or sectioning of teeth has been described in Chapter 13.

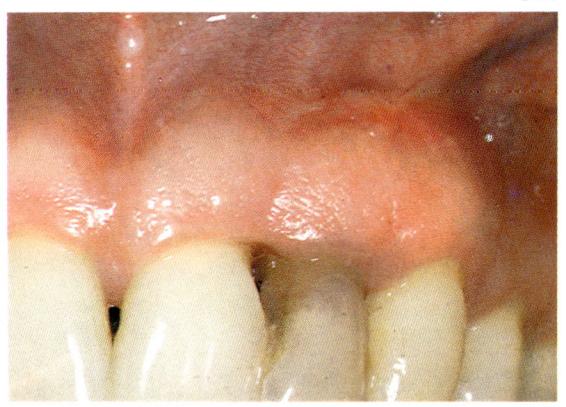

The sequence of treatment

321. When the treatment plan for a patient necessitates a multi-disciplined approach the correct sequence of the various components is crucial to the success of the whole (see Appendix 4). This patient has chronic periodontitis with approximately 2–3mm of interproximal bone destruction.

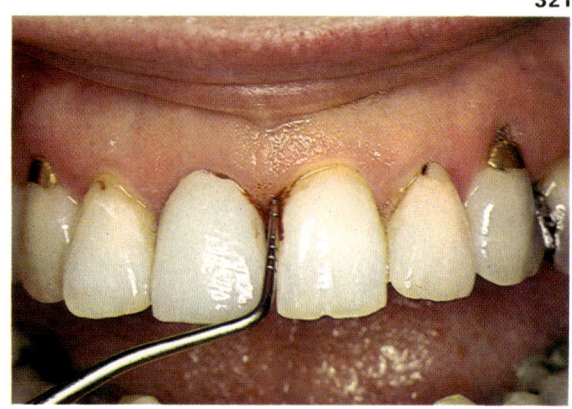

322. The upper right lateral incisor has begun to migrate labially. This appears to be due to forces exerted by the tongue and lower lip. The initial phase of therapy has included oral hygiene instruction, and scaling and polishing of the teeth. The patient has achieved good plaque control.

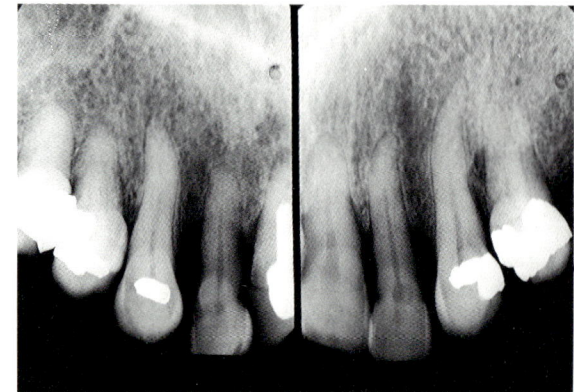

323. The upper right lateral incisor is being realigned with a simple orthodontic appliance.

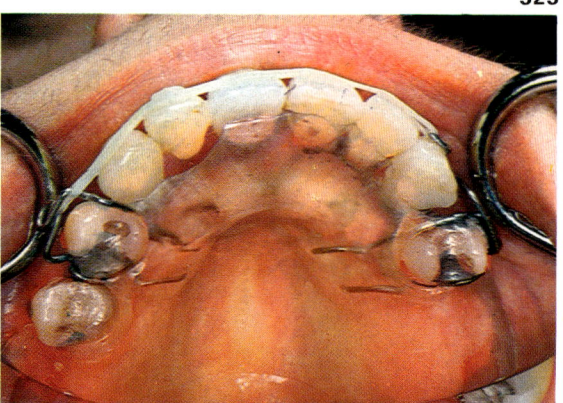

324. There are still periodontal pockets present and these are being eliminated by means of an inverse bevel flap procedure.

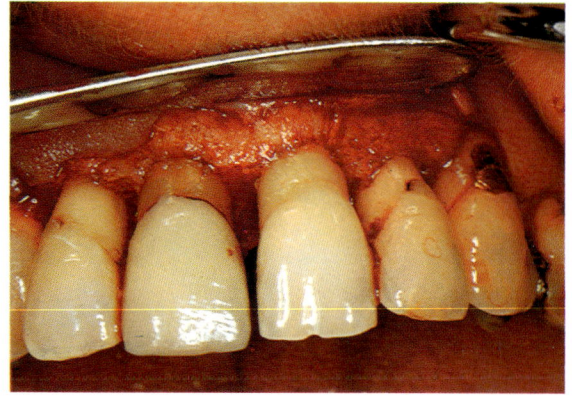

The sequence of treatment

325. The flap has been repositioned apically and sutured. The level of the margins of the flap should be compared with the level of the gingival margin in **321** to enable the degree of apical repositioning to be assessed.

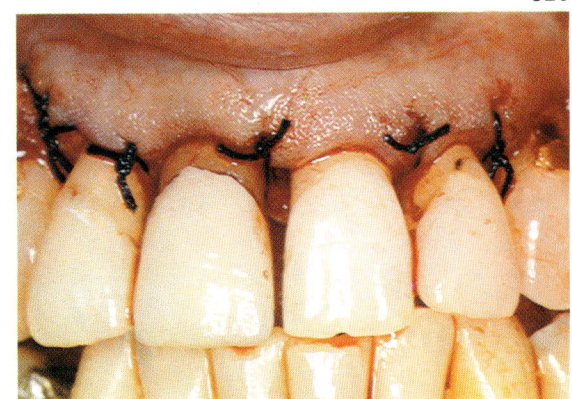

326. Porcelain bonded to gold crowns have been fitted. The distal abutment teeth on either side have reduced alveolar bone support as a result of the previous periodontal disease. Splinting was used to provide paired abutment teeth and thereby to distribute the torque produced by the free end saddle prosthesis. The right lateral incisor is splinted to provide permanent retention after the orthodontic treatment, and to prevent recurrence of migration.

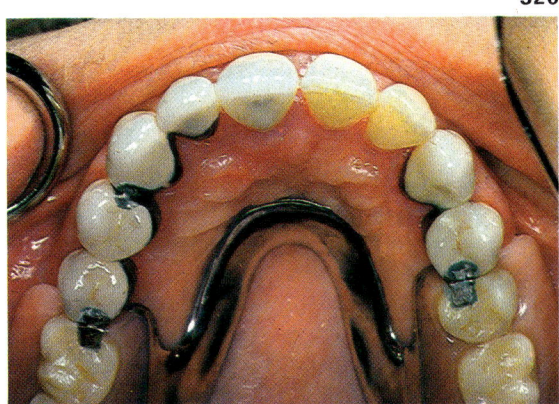

Appendix 1

Aetiology and pathology of periodontal disease

Initiating factors

Plaque formation
Salivary mucin
Microorganisms
Substrate

Metabolites from plaque microorganisms
Endotoxins
Enzymes
Antigens
Other chemical agents

Host response

Inflammation
Vascular response
Cellular exudate

Humoural immune response
Antibodies to toxins, enzymes, other antigens
Antibody + Antigen → Complex

Activation of complement
(By complex or endotoxins)
Enhances phagocytosis
Generates anaphylactic factor
Results in cell lysis

Cellular immune response
Inhibits macrophage migration
Inhibits migration of mononuclear cells
Causes lysis of sensitised cells
Activates osteoclasts

Factors which aid retention of plaque

Inadequate cleaning
Calculus
Deposits from tobacco smoke
Iatrogenic factors

Local protective mechanisms

Saliva
Dento-gingival form
Attachment of junctional epithelium
Epithelial cell turnover
Crevicular fluid

Factors which interfere with host response

Systemic diseases
Blood dyscrasias
Collagen disorders

Congenital defects
Papillon Lefèvre
Mongolism

Drugs
Hydantoin
Immuno-suppressive drugs
Contraceptive hormones

Hormonal changes
Puberty
Pregnancy
Menopause
Diabetes

Appendix 2 — Periodontal indices

Epidemiological studies of periodontal disease have been carried out on a variety of population groups. Clinical epidemiology has also been used to assess periodontal treatment procedures. This work has been made possible by the development of periodontal indices. These indices consist of a series of definitions designed to measure the status of the periodontium and/or the associated aetiological agents. A selection of the more commonly used indices is presented below:

The Periodontal Index
Russell 1956

0. There is neither overt inflammation in the investing tissue nor loss of function due to destruction of supporting tissue. Radiographic appearance is normal.

1. Mild gingivitis. There is an overt area of inflammation in the free gingiva but this area does not circumscribe the tooth.

2. Gingivitis. Inflammation completely circumscribes the tooth, but there is no apparent break in the epithelial attachment.

4. (Not used in field studies.) There is an early notch-like resorption of the alveolar crest.

6. Gingivitis with pocket formation. The epithelial attachment has been broken and there is a pocket (not merely a deepened gingival crevice due to swelling in the free gingiva).
There is no interference with normal masticatory function, the tooth is firm in its socket and has not drifted.
Radiographically there is bone loss involving the entire alveolar crest up to half of the length of the tooth root (distance from apex to cemento-enamel junction).

8. Advanced destruction with loss of masticatory function. The tooth may be loose, may have drifted, may sound dull on percussion with a metallic instrument, may be depressible in its socket.
Radiographically there is advanced bone loss involving more than one-half of the length of the tooth root, or a definite widening of the periodontal membrane. There may be root resorption or rarefaction at the apex.

RULE: When in doubt assign the lesser score.

The Gingival Index
Löe and Silness 1963

0. Normal gingiva.

1. Mild inflammation, slight change in colour, slight oedema, no bleeding on probing.

2. Moderate inflammation, redness, oedema and glazing. Bleeding on probing.

3. Severe inflammation, marked redness and oedema, ulceration. Tendency to spontaneous haemorrhage.

The Plaque Index
Silness and Löe 1964

0. No plaque.

1. Film of plaque, visible only by removal on probe or by disclosing.

2. Moderate accumulation of deposits within the pockets or on the margins which can be seen with the naked eye.

3. Heavy accumulation of soft material filling the niche between gingival margin and tooth surface. Interdental region is filled with debris.

The Oral Hygiene Index
Greene and Vermillion 1960

0. No debris or stain.

1. Soft debris covering not more than one-third of tooth surface.

2. Soft debris covering more than one-third but not more than two-thirds of tooth surface.

3. Soft debris covering over two-thirds of tooth surface.

Appendix 3   Periodontal assessment form

The use of an assessment form as illustrated facilitates both documenting of the patient's history and recording of the clinical examination. The form is useful for the assistant when taking notes, and the layout presents the case record under clear headings. The incorporated grid may be used for recording pockets and the mobility of teeth. There are four segments for recording pockets at the mesial, mid-facial, distal and mid-lingual of each tooth.

For the more complex case the periodontal chart may be used (see second illustration). This chart is of particular benefit if completed prior to embarking on the more advanced stages of treatment. The residual pockets should be marked on the chart and these can then be related to the anatomy of the soft tissues and to the radiographic picture. Charting also enables the distribution of the pathology to be related to local plaque retaining factors. Where periodontal surgery is indicated the planning of the order of treatment is facilitated by having the distribution of the pockets presented graphically.

The outline chart is presented in this appendix so that copies may be taken for clinical use.

PERIODONTAL ASSESSMENT FORM   DATE

NAME   **DATE OF BIRTH**

ADDRESS

COMPLAINT

HISTORY OF COMPLAINT

ORAL HISTORY

ORAL HYGIENE METHODS

MEDICAL HISTORY

SOCIAL HISTORY

EXTRA ORAL EXAMINATION

INTRA ORAL EXAMINATION – MUCOSA

FRENAE

MARGINAL GINGIVAE

PAPILLAE

ATTACHED GINGIVAE

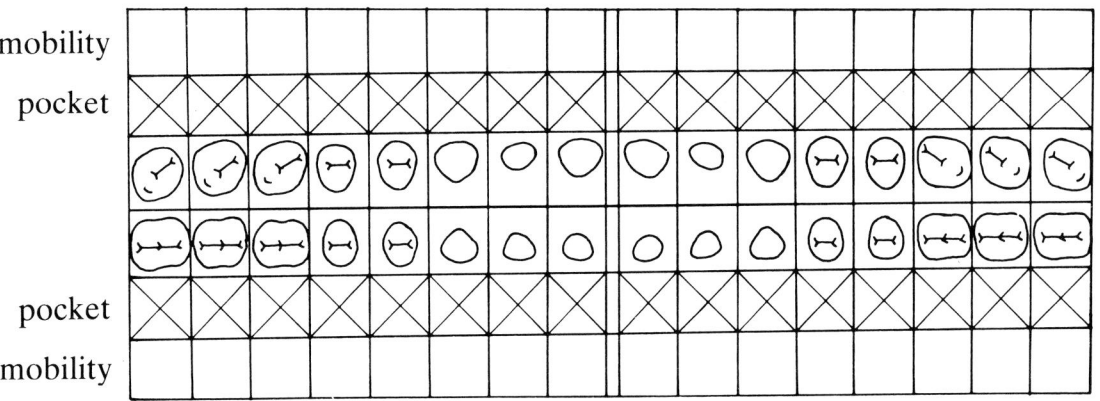

PLAQUE

CALCULUS – SUPRA GINGIVAL

        SUB GINGIVAL

OCCLUSION

RADIOGRAPHIC ASSESSMENT

SUMMARY – DIAGNOSIS AND AETIOLOGY

TREATMENT PLAN

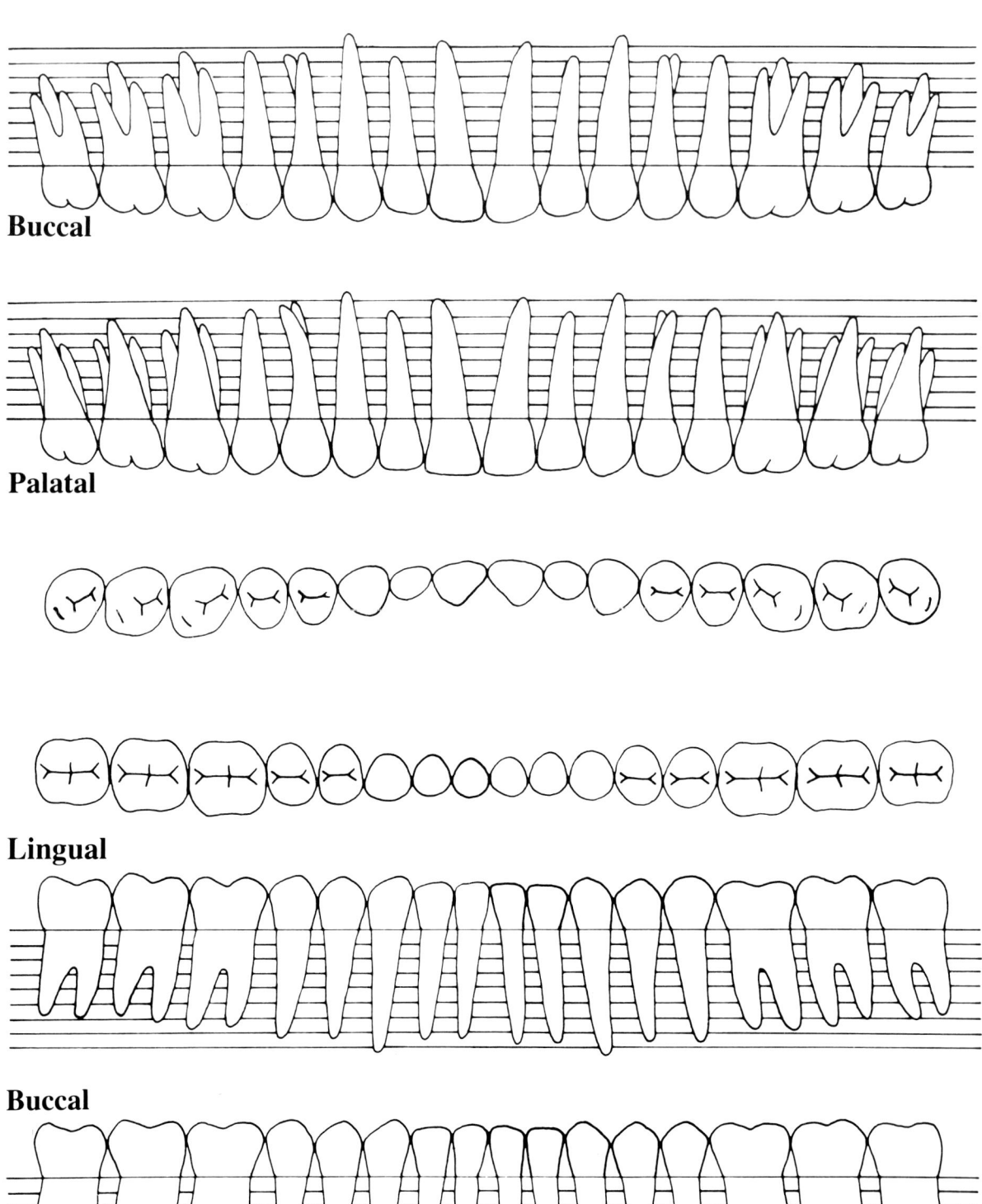

Buccal

Palatal

Lingual

Buccal

120

Appendix 4

Sequence for the components of treatment

Initial therapy
(a) Oral hygiene instruction.
(b) Scaling and polishing.
(c) Occlusal adjustment.
(d) Smoothing margins of restorations.
(e) Replacing unsatisfactory plastic restorations.
(f) Extractions.
(g) Temporary prosthesis.

Advanced therapy
(a) Orthodontic treatment.
(b) Periodontal surgery.
(c) Advanced restorative procedures.
(d) Prosthetic reconstruction.

N.B. The various components of treatment may be transposed where this is indicated but in general the procedures in the second group should not be undertaken until those in the first group have been completed. Periodontal surgery should precede advanced restorative procedures, as the margins of the restorations should be planned in relation to a stabilised gingival level.

Maintenance
On completion of therapy regular recall appointments must be arranged in order that the motivation of the patient can be reinforced and the importance of continued plaque control can be stressed.

Appendix 5

Management of the surgical patient

Preparation of the patient

It is essential that the patient be fully informed about the aims and objectives of the operation prior to surgery. They must also be warned about any disadvantages which can be anticipated, for example the likelihood of subsequent recession and the possibility of hypersensitivity to heat and to cold. The latter is generally only a temporary phenomenon provided that plaque control is maintained.

The operative procedure

Periodontal surgery is generally carried out under local analgesia. For the apprehensive patient this may be augmented with intravenous sedation (Ruggerio 1975) or relative analgesia (Shane 1975). Where handicapped patients are to be treated or where it is planned to undertake surgery on extensive areas at one visit, then hospitalisation and the use of general anaesthesia may be indicated.

Periodontal surgery is usually planned so that the mouth can be treated in segments, allowing one region to heal before progressing to the next. This enables the operator to decide the extent of the area to be undertaken at one visit, according to the complexity of the procedure. Other factors will also influence the planning of surgery, including the experience of the operator and the requirements of the patient. The use of sedation or general anaesthesia may enable a larger area to be undertaken, or perhaps all the treatment to be completed, at one session. It is comparatively rare for a patient after completion of plaque control treatment to require periodontal surgery involving all the teeth.

The diagrams illustrate the more common methods of treating the mouth segmentally:

(A) The division of the mouth into six segments provides relatively small areas to be treated surgically at each visit; this is of benefit when surgery is relatively complicated.

(B) The undertaking of treatment in quarterly divisions results in fewer surgical visits. After surgery there is often a difference in the levels of the gingival margins between the operated and unoperated segments. Terminating periodontal surgery at the midline may result in this stepped effect being visible, at least until the neighbouring segment has been treated.

(C), (D) and (E) Further reductions in the number of surgical visits may be achieved by dividing the mouth into thirds or halves. If possible the treatment should be designed so that the patient has at least one segment of the mouth not involved by surgery, which he can use for eating.

Postoperative medication

The amount of pain after periodontal surgery is variable (Strahan and Glenwright 1967). Postoperatively the patient can be given 1000mg of paracetemol or similar analgesic by mouth, and this dose may be repeated every six hours.

Postoperative infection is rare after periodontal surgery, and in general antibiotic cover is not indicated. The use of antibiotics, however, is necessary where there is a medical indication, for example a history of rheumatic fever.

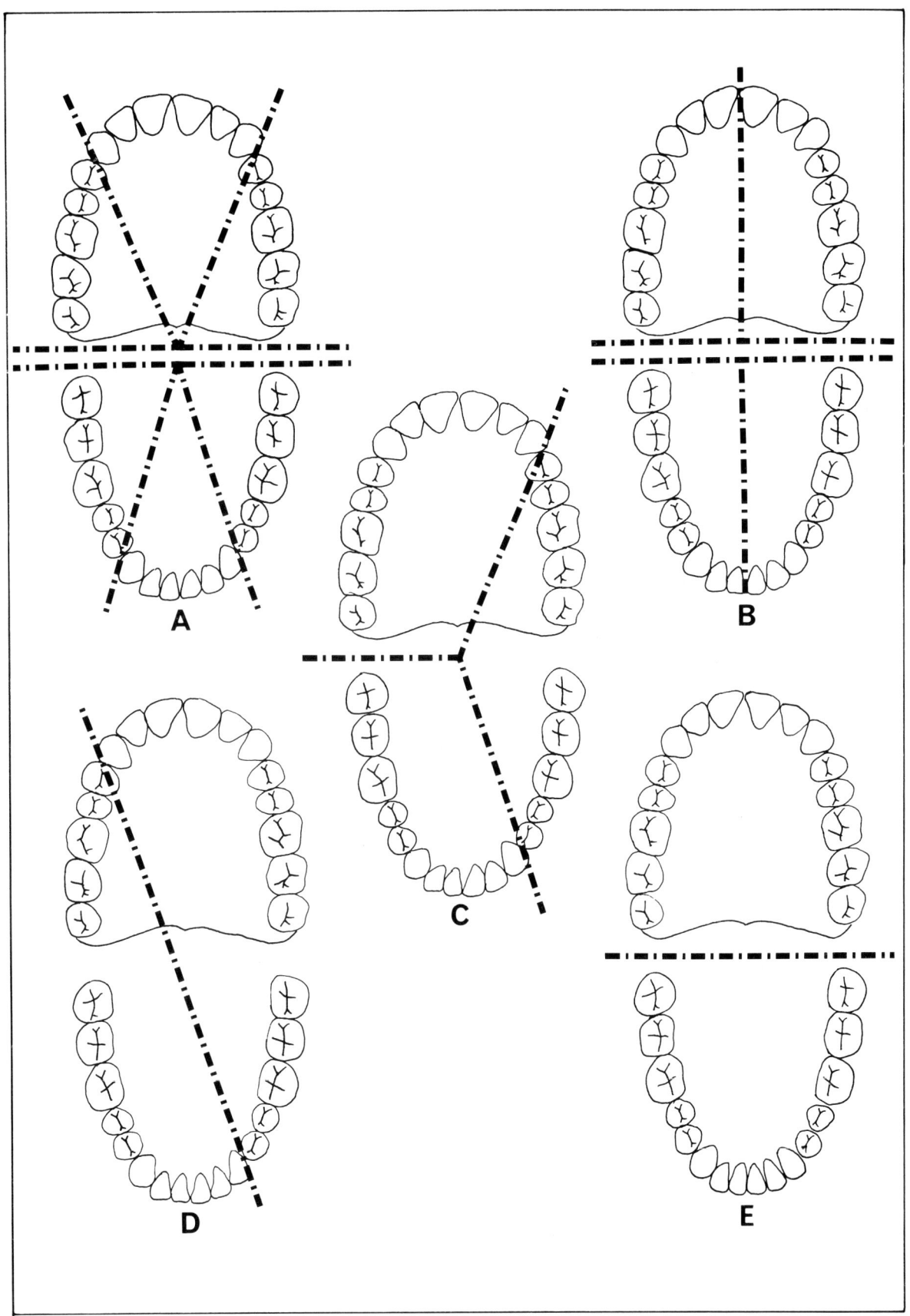

Postoperative care

The patient should be given instructions about postoperative care. These are given verbally but may also be reinforced by printed instructions which should provide the following information:

Instructions for the week following periodontal surgery

1. If you have pain following periodontal surgery, take analgesic tablets such as paracetamol or aspirin in the dose advised by the manufacturer.

2. You may have had antibiotics prescribed; if so you should take these as directed until the course of antibiotics has been completed.

3. If dressings have been applied these should remain in place until your next appointment. If any of the dressing comes away during the first two days or if the exposed area is painful or bleeds, you should return for treatment.

4. There may be a minor amount of bleeding from the surgical site for the first day, but this should soon stop. Persistence of bleeding is uncommon but can usually be controlled by the application of firm pressure to the area with a finger covered with a few layers of gauze or similar material. If the bleeding is severe or persists, or if there is undue swelling, you should return for treatment.

5. Clean the unoperated regions of your mouth as usual.

6. The surgically treated area should be cleaned with a mouthwash. A salt solution may be used – add two teaspoonfuls of salt to half a glass of water. Alternatively you may have been given an antiseptic mouthwash to use.

7. Strenuous exercise, smoking and alcohol should be avoided for the first few days after surgery. Avoid eating hard, spicy or sticky foods during the week after surgery. Try to eat only on teeth not in the operated area.

Care during the second week after surgery

1. In those areas of the mouth which have not been treated surgically, use your normal cleaning methods.

2. Clean the surgical area both with the toothbrush and between the teeth, using the methods you have been shown but with slightly less force to avoid damaging the healing gum.

3. Use a mouthwash if one has been prescribed.

Long-term care

1. Within about two weeks after surgery, cleaning procedures should be resumed using the normal amount of pressure. Both toothbrushing and cleaning between the teeth must be performed thoroughly, and this routine must be continued in the future.

2. Attend your dentist regularly for routine examination and care. Regular examinations are essential to make sure that the inflammation of the gum does not recur.

Appendix 6 — Local analgesia in periodontal therapy

Choice of analgesic

The analgesic preparation in general use for dental procedures is 2% lignocaine with adrenaline 1 in 80,000. This is available in cartridges which usually contain 2 ml of the solution, although other capacities are available. Injection of solution into a blood vessel can be avoided by using an aspirating syringe.

Alternative analgesic preparations have been developed, for example 3% prilocaine with felypressin 0.03 units per ml. These are of value for the treatment of patients who might react adversely to the lignocaine with adrenaline preparation. For example an analgesic solution which does not contain adrenaline is preferable for patients with cardiovascular disease, hypertension, hyperthyroidism or who are taking tricyclic antidepressants. The disadvantage of the prilocaine with felypressin preparation is that haemorrhage control is not as good (Newcomb and Waite 1972).

Injection sites for local analgesia

It has been shown by Hecht and App (1974) that local infiltration of analgesic provides better control of haemorrhage during periodontal surgery than the use of nerve block analgesia. To reduce pain as few injection sites as possible should be used to achieve initial analgesia. On the facial aspect after the initial penetration of the mucosa the needle is advanced horizontally through the tissues at the level of the apices of the teeth (**148**). Analgesic solution is slowly injected ahead of the needle. Three injection sites are usually required for each quadrant on the vestibular aspect. On the palatal and lingual aspects the analgesic solution is infiltrated at strategic points in relation to the nerve supply of the area.

When initial analgesia has been obtained further solution is infiltrated into the papilla and the marginal gingiva associated with each tooth. This reinforces the analgesia and results in further vasoconstriction (**149**).

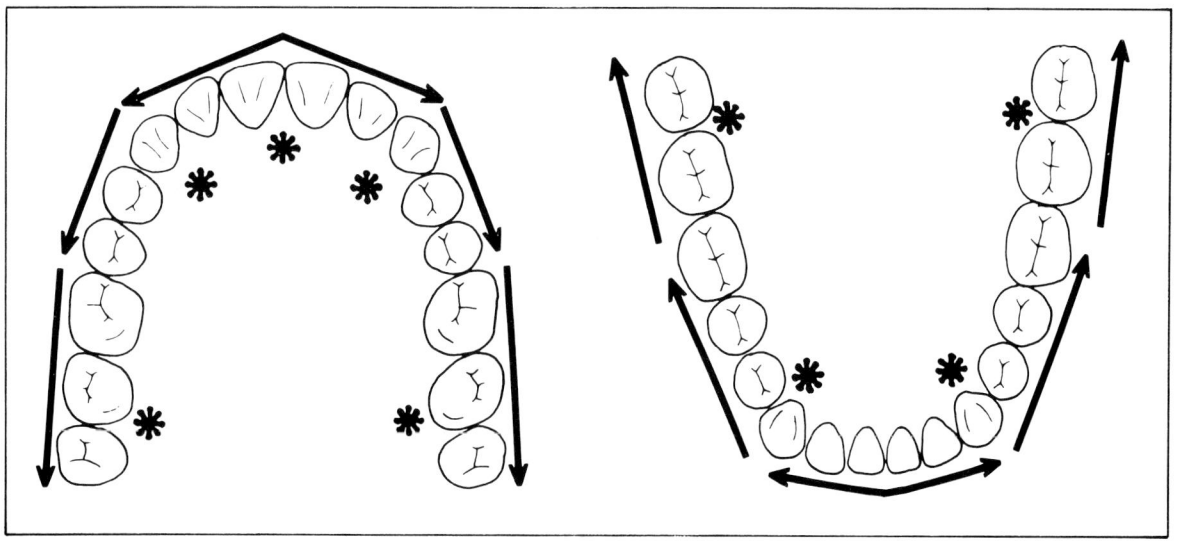

Appendix 7

Instrumentation for periodontal surgery

It is convenient to assemble the basic instruments for periodontal surgery as a standardised kit and after sterilisation this can be stored ready for use. The kit should be designed so that it comprises the basic instruments required for the more common surgical procedures. Instruments which are used only rarely may be kept separately in individual sterile containers. The advantage of this system is that it avoids the need for different instrument packages for each type of surgical procedure.

Sterile drapes should be available with the surgical set-up on which to lay out the instruments and with which to cover the patient's chest. Sufficient sterile towels should also be provided for both the operator and assistant to dry their hands before and during the procedure.

The second illustration shows accessory equipment which may be required during the course of periodontal surgery.

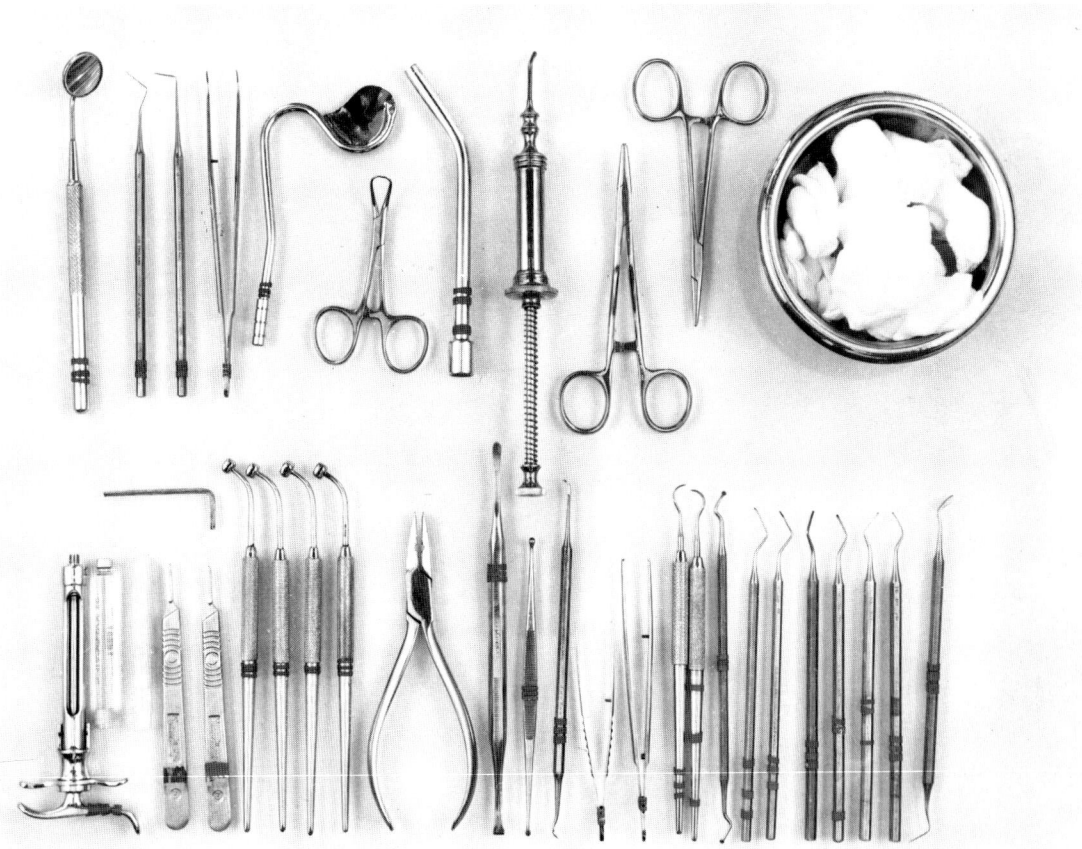

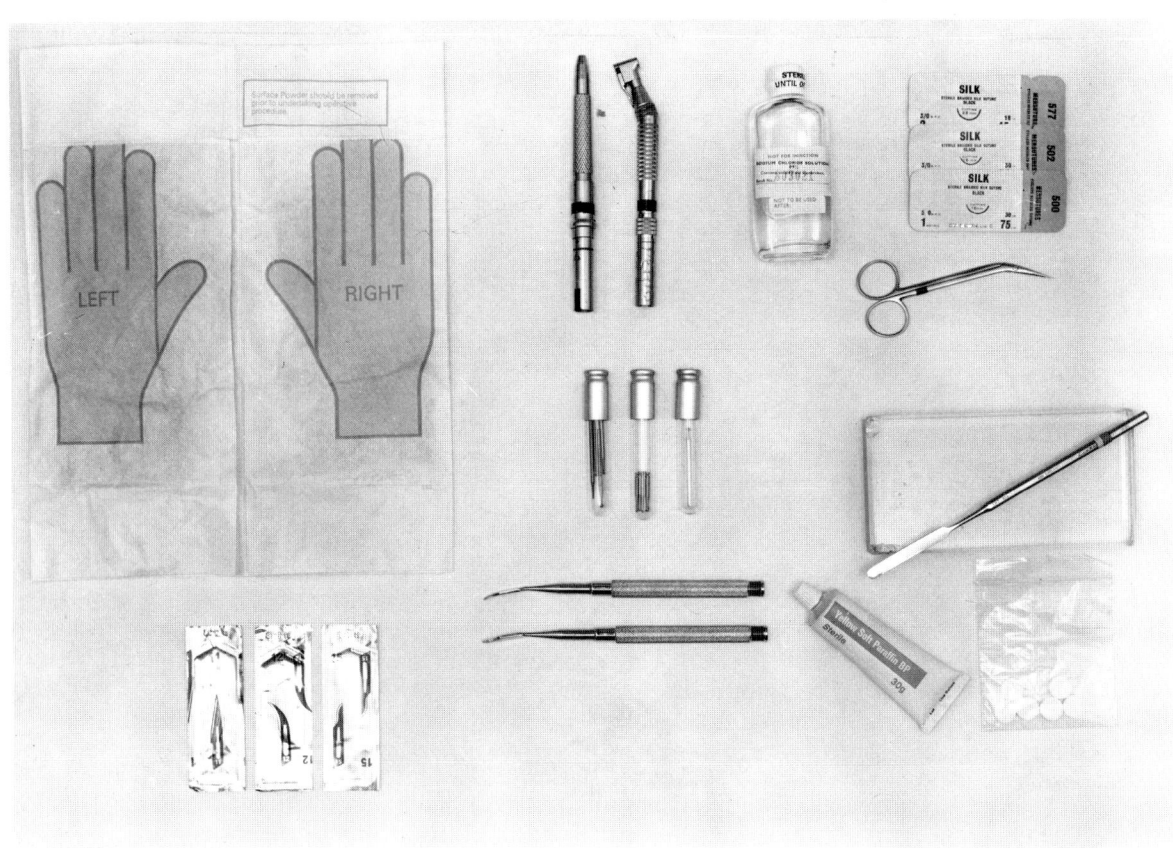

Appendix 8 Periodontal bone defects

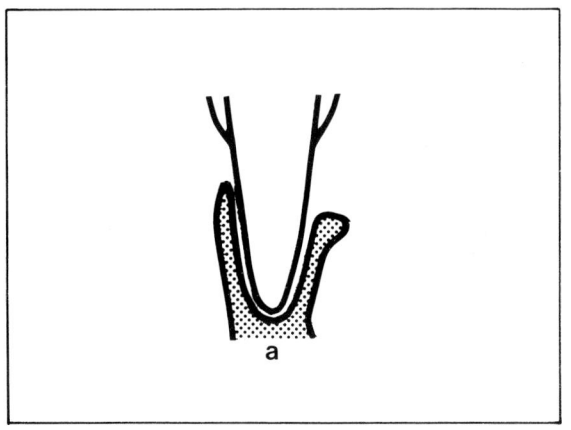

(a) Exostoses. Marginal exostoses may be caused by an alteration in the balance between bone resorption and bone deposition as a result of chronic inflammation.

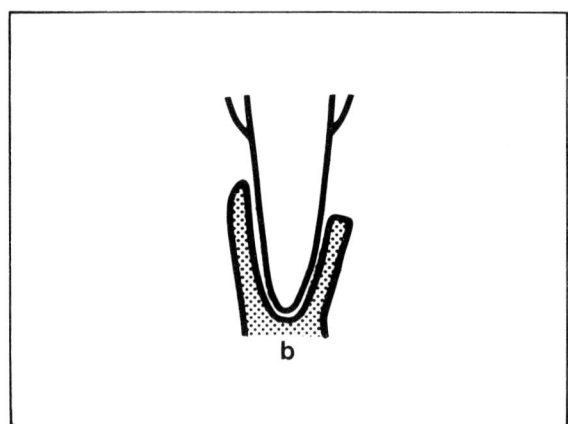

(b) Ledge. Ledging of the marginal bone results when there is a loss in height of bone without an accompanying reduction in thickness.

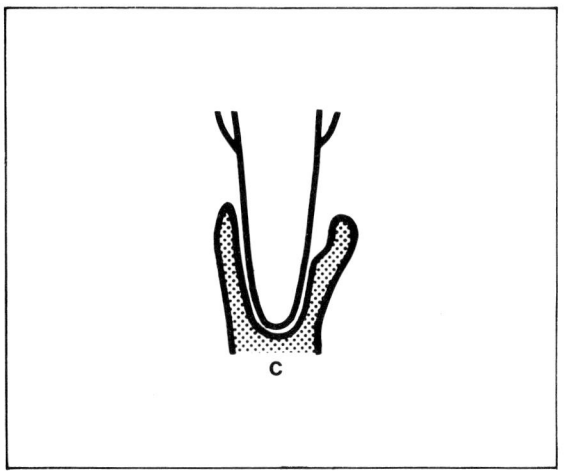

(c) Ditching. Ditching is a type of one wall defect (as "f") and may involve several aspects of the tooth.

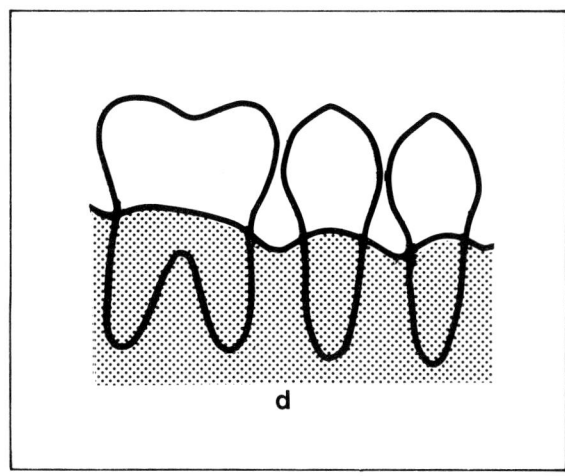

(d) Reverse architecture. Reverse architecture results when there is a more rapid rate of resorption of the interproximal bone than marginal bone.

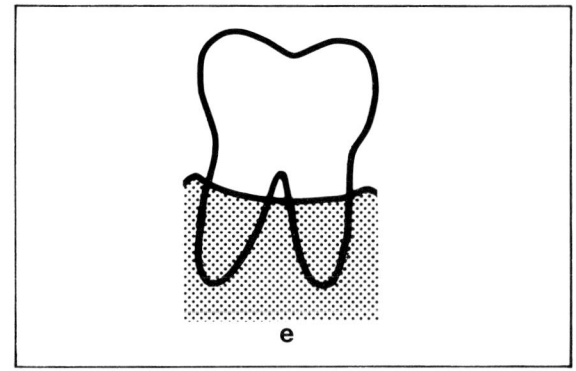

(e) Furcation involvement. On multirooted teeth bone loss from periodontal disease may result in exposure of the furcation regions.

(f), (g) The one-walled bony defect. Infra-bony defects are classified by the number of bony walls present. The one-walled defect may occur as in *(f)* or alternatively as a hemi-septal defect *(g)*.

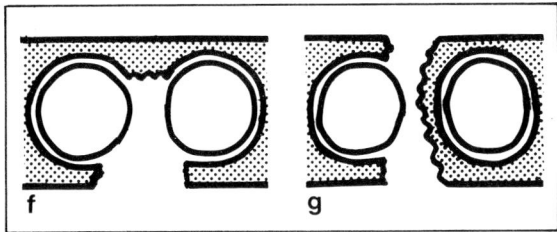

(h), (i) The two-walled bony defect. The two-walled defect may be seen as in *(h)* or alternatively as a crater *(i)*.

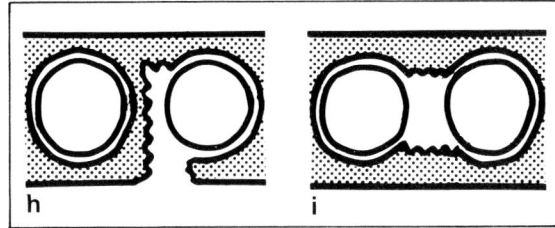

(j) The three-walled defect. The three-walled defect is illustrated in *(j)*.

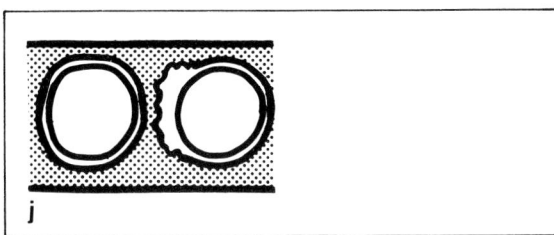

Frequently the anatomy of bony defects is complicated. They may involve several aspects of the tooth, and may commence as three-walled, becoming two-walled and finally end up as one-walled defects at their coronal extremity.

Appendix 9 — Periodontal suturing techniques

The objectives of interproximal suturing are to prevent the flap being displaced apically and to obtain adaptation of the flap to the underlying tissues. (a) Interrupted sutures are used when it is required to secure the buccal and palatal papillae under equal tension across the interproximal spaces. (b) The sling suture is used to suspend adjoining papillae without involving the papillae on the opposite aspect of the teeth. (c) The continuous suture is used to suspend the papillae of several consecutive teeth. It can be used for securing a buccal flap which has been used in conjunction with a palatal gingivectomy. The continuous suture is also useful for securing buccal and palatal flaps under independent tensions. For example, the buccal flap may be sutured relatively loosely to permit it to be repositioned apically. The palatal flap which is to be replaced is then sutured under slight tension.

The flap must also be stabilised against movement in a coronal direction. The position of the flap at the relieving incision is determined by the placement of the lateral suture. Maximum apical movement is achieved by placing the suture through the papilla on the flap and at the muco-gingival junction on the unoperated tissue. Where there is difficulty in maintaining the flap in the correct relationship a periosteal suture may be used. The suture is passed through the mucosa of the vestibule and into the underlying periosteum. It is then brought out again through the mucosa and tied. This is a difficult technique, and in some regions of the mouth the periosteum is not thick enough to permit a suture to be placed.

The most common method of providing resistance to coronal movement of the flap is by careful placement of a periodontal dressing. For a repositioned flap the material should be of firm consistency when placed so that it has sufficient body to control the flap. Retention of the dressing is obtained by applying pressure over each interproximal region to obtain adaptation.

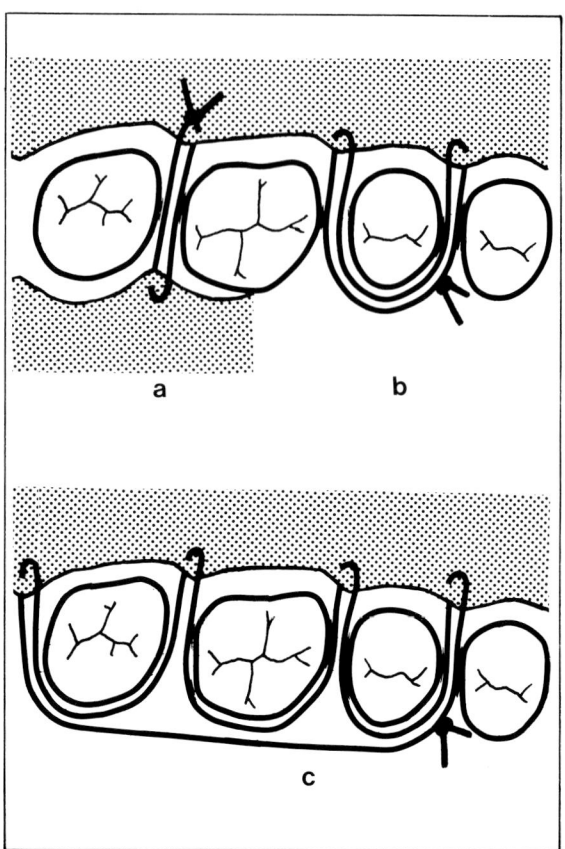

Appendix 10 Wound healing

Gingivectomy (Chapter 11)

(a) The first stage in healing after gingivectomy is the formation of a blood clot over the wound surface.

(b) During the first two weeks after surgery granulation tissue forms within the clot, and epithelium from the wound edges migrates over this granulation tissue.

(c) From about day 10 to about day 30 there is organisation of connective tissue and keratinization of epithelium. During this period a new junctional epithelium and gingival sulcus develop (Stahl *et al* 1972).

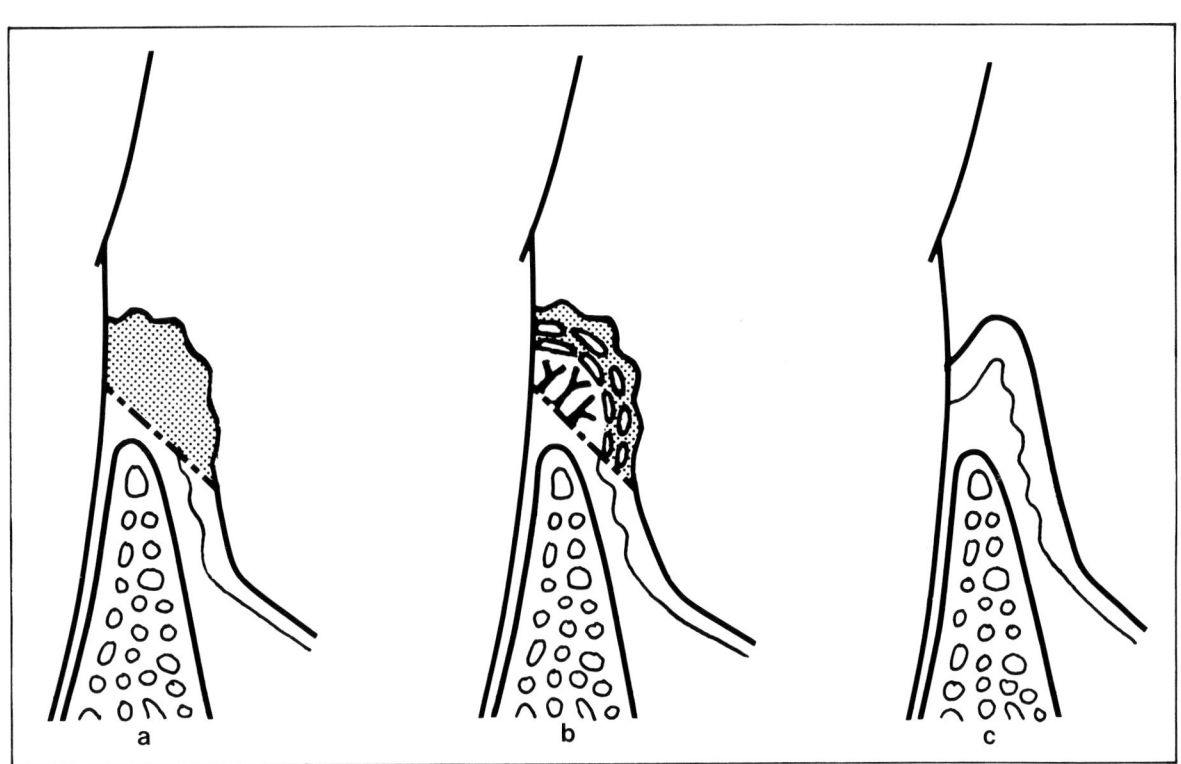

Periodontal flap surgery (Chapter 12)
(a) The initial phase in the healing process after periodontal flap surgery is clot formation between the flap and the underlying tissue.

(b) In the first two weeks postoperatively granulation tissue develops within the clot. Near the surface of the clot the space between the flap and the tooth is rapidly bridged by the migration of epithelial cells.

(b) and (c) The exposure of alveolar bone at the time of flap surgery results in subsequent resorption; this takes place mainly during the first three weeks after the operation.

The amount of net bone loss depends on several factors, for example on the thickness of the marginal bone, on whether bone surgery is performed, and on whether the alveolar bone is completely covered with the flap after surgery or whether a width of marginal bone is left exposed. Studies on human subjects indicate that there is a loss of 0.5–1mm when bone is covered (Donnenfield et al 1964). At the other extreme there is severe and prolonged resorption of bone following denudation procedures in which bone is left exposed after surgery (Costitch and Ramfjord 1968b).

(d) Towards the end of the initial three week period deposition of bone commences and this continues for 10 weeks or more after surgery. As a result there is a partial restoration of the lost bone (Costitch and Ramfjord 1968a).

The organisation of the connective tissue, and the reformation of the junctional epithelium and gingival sulcus take place during the period between approximately day 10 and day 40.

Induction of keratinization in epithelium
One of the aims of muco-gingival procedures is to achieve a functional zone of keratinized gingiva. The techniques which have been described in Chapters 12, 15 and 16 have achieved the required zone of keratinized tissue by relocating existing gingival tissue. It has been demonstrated by several workers that the stimuli causing epithelium to keratinize originate in the underlying connective tissue (Heaney 1974, Karring et al 1975). The principles of muco-gingival procedures are based on the conservation and relocation of existing keratinized tissue, including the underlying corium, so that the resultant epithelium is induced to keratinize.

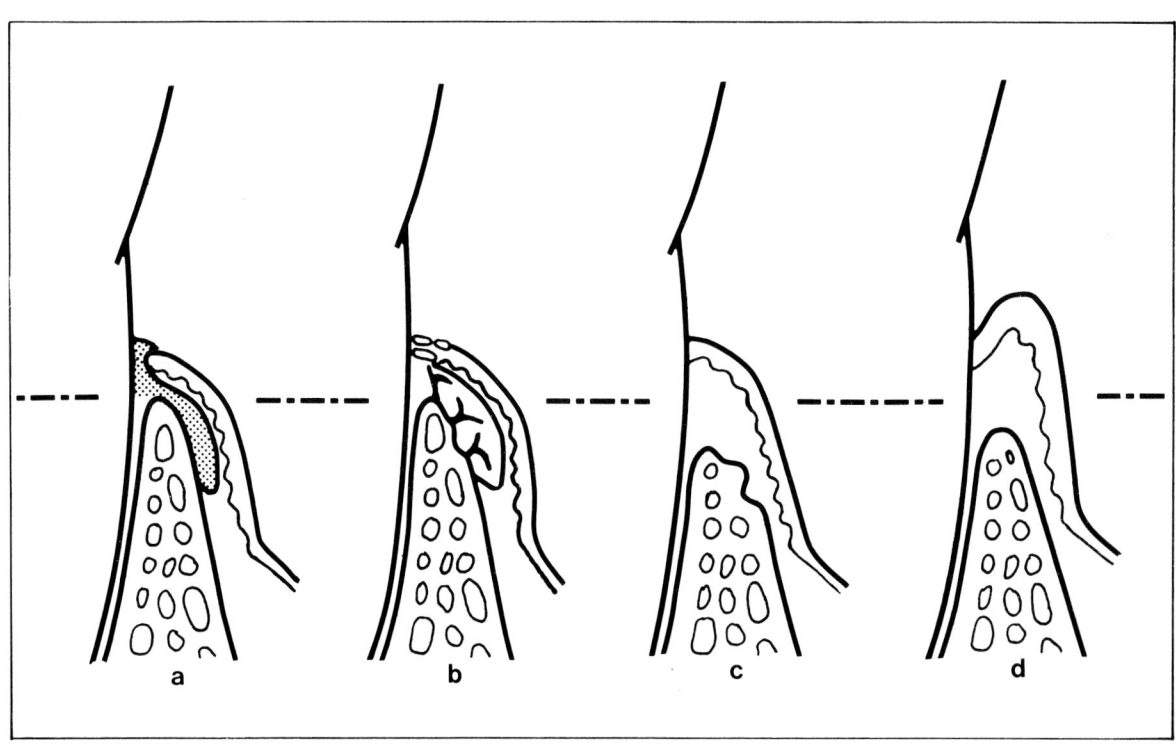

Bibliography

Ainamo, J. and Löe, H. (1966). Anatomical characteristics of gingiva – a clinical and microscopic study of free and attached gingiva. *J. Periodontol.*, **37**, 5.

Ainamo, J. (1972). Relationship between malalignment of teeth and periodontal disease. *Scand. J. Dent. Res.*, **80**, 104.

Aleo, J. J., De Renzis, F. A., Farber, P. A. and Varboncoeur, A. P. (1974). The presence and biologic activity of cementum-bound endotoxin. *J. Periodontol.*, **45**, 672.

Arno, A., Waerhaug, J., Lovdal, A. and Schei, O. (1958). Incidence of gingivitis as related to sex, occupation, tobacco consumption, toothbrushing, and age. *Oral Surg., Oral Med. and Oral Path.*, **11**, 587.

Arno, A., Schei, O., Lovdal, A. and Waerhaug, J. (1959). Alveolar bone loss as a function of tobacco consumption. *Acta Odontol. Scand.*, **17**, 3.

Attström, R. (1970). Presence of leukocytes in crevices of healthy and chronically inflamed gingivae. *J. Periodontol. Res.*, **5**, 42.

Baer, P. N. (1971). The case for periodontosis as a clinical entity. *J. Periodontol.*, **42**, 516.

Bang, J., Cimasoni, G., Rosenbusch, C. and Duckert, A. (1973). Sodium, potassium and calcium contents of crevicular exudate: their relations to gingivitis and periodontitis. *J. Periodontol.*, **44**, 770.

Bergenholtz, A. (1972). Mechanical cleaning in oral hygiene. *Oral Hygiene* – Copenhagen: Munksgaard, Publishers.

Bergenholtz, A., Bjorne, A. and Vikström, G. (1974). The plaque-removing ability of some common interdental aids. *J. Clin. Periodont.*, **1**, 160.

Bergman, B., Hugoson, A. and Olsson, C. (1971). Periodontal and prosthetic conditions in patients treated with removable partial dentures and artificial crowns. A longitudinal two year study. *Acta Odontol. Scand.*, **29**, 621.

Bernimoulin, J. P., Lüscher, B. and Mühlemann, H. R. (1975). Coronally repositioned periodontal flap. *J. Clin. Periodont.*, **2**, 1.

Bowers, G. M. (1963). A study of the width of attached gingiva. *J. Periodontol.*, **34**, 201.

Brady, J. M., Gray, W. A. and Bhaskar, S. M. (1973). Electron microscope study of the effect of water jet lavage devices on dental plaque. *J. Dent. Res.*, **52**, 1310.

Caffesse, R. G. and Nasjleti, C. E. (1976). Enzymatic penetration through intact sulcular epithelium. *J. Periodontol.*, **47**, 391.

Chase, R. (1974). Subgingival curettage in periodontal therapy. *J. Periodontol.*, **45**, 107.

Ciancio, G. S. and Nisengard, R. J. (1975). Resins in periodontal splinting. *Dent. Clin. N. Amer.*, **19**, 235, Apr.

Clark, J. W., Weatherford, T. W. and Mann, W. V. (1969). The wire ligature acrylic splint. *J. Periodontol.*, **40**, 371.

Cohen, D. W., Friedman, L. A., Shapiro, J., Kyle, G. C. and Franklin, S. (1970). Diabetes and periodontal disease: two year longitudinal observations. *J. Periodontol.*, **41**, 709.

Cohen, D. W. Friedman, L., Shapiro, J. and Kyle, G. C. (1971). A longitudinal investigation of the periodontal changes during pregnancy II. *J. Periodontol.*, **42**, 653.

Costitch, E. R. and Ramfjord, S. P. (1968a). Healing after partial denudation of the alveolar process. *J. Periodontol.*, **39**, 127.

Costitch, E. R. and Ramfjord, S. P. (1968b). Healing after periosteal exposure. *J. Periodontol.*, **39**, 199.

Cox, M. O., Crawford, J. J., Lundblad, R. L. and McFall, W. T. (1974). Oral leucocytes and gingivitis in the primary dentition. *J. Periodont. Res.*, **9**, 23.

Crawford, A., Socransky, S. S. and Bratthal, G. (1975). Predominant cultivable microbiota of advanced periodontitis. *J. Dent. Res.*, **54**, A.A.D.R. Abstract 209.

Donnenfield, O. W., Marks, R. and Glickman, I. (1964). The apically respositioned flap. *J. Periodontol.*, **35**, 381.

Donnenfield, O. W., Stanley, H. R. and Bagdonoff, L. (1974). A nine-month clinical and histological study of patients on diphenylhydantoin following gingivectomy. *J. Periodontol.*, **45**, 547.

Dordick, B., Coslet, J. G. and Seibert, J. S. (1976). Clinical evaluation of free autogenous gingival grafts placed on alveolar bone. *J. Periodontol.*, **47**, 559.

Douglas, G. L. (1976). Mucogingival repairs in periodontal surgery. *Dent. Clin. N. Amer.*, **20**, Jan., 107.

Duckworth, R., Waterhouse, J. P., Britton, D. E. R., Nuki, K., Sheiham, A., Winter, R. and Blake, C. G. (1966). Acute ulcerative gingivitis. *Brit. Dent. J.*, **120**, 599.

Ellegaard, B. (1976). Bone grafts in periodontal attachment procedures. *J. Clin. Periodont.*, **3**, No.5 (Extra Issue).

Ellegaard, B. and Löe, H. (1971). New attachment of periodontal tissue after treatment of intra-bony lesions. *J. Periodontol.*, **42**, 648.

Epstein, S. and Scopp, I. W. (1977). Antibiotics and the intra-oral abscess. *J. Periodontol.*, **48**, 236.

Folke, L. E. A. and Stallard, R. E. (1967). Periodontal microcirculation as revealed by plastic microspheres. *J. Periodont. Res.*, **2**, 53.

Frank, A. L. (1967). Improvement of the crown-root ratio – endodontic implants. *J. Am. Dent. Assoc.*, **74**, 451.

Friedman, N. (1962). Mucogingival surgery: the apically repositioned flap. *J. Periodontol.*, **33**, 328.

Geering, A. H. (1974). Occlusal interferences and functional disturbances of the masticatory system. *J. Clin. Periodont.*, **1**, 112.

Genco, R. J., Mashimo, P. A., Krygier, G. and Ellison, S. A. (1974). Antibody-mediated effects on the periodontium. *J. Periodontol.*, **45**, 330.

Gibbons, R. J. and Van Houte, J. (1973). On the formation of dental plaques. *J. Periodontol.*, **44**, 347.

Gilmore, N. and Sheiham, A. (1971). Overhanging dental restorations and periodontal disease. *J. Periodontol.*, **42**, 8.

Glickman, I. (1972). *Clinical periodontology*. Philadelphia: W. B. Saunders.

Glickman, I. and Smulow, J. B. (1969). The combined effects of inflammation and trauma from occlusion. *Int. Dent. J.*, **19**, 393.

Goldman, H. M. (1951). Gingivectomy. *Oral Surg., Oral Med. and Oral Path.*, **4**, 1136.

Grant, D. and Bernick, S. (1972). The periodontium of ageing individuals. *J. Periodontol.*, **43**, 660.

Greene, J. C. (1960). Periodontal disease in India: report of an epidemiological study. *J. Dent. Res.*, **39**, 302.

Greene, J. C. and Vermillion, J. R. (1960). The oral hygiene index. *J. Am. Dent. Assoc.*, **61**, 172.

Greene, J. C. and Vermillion, J. R. (1963). The effects of controlled oral hygiene on the human adult periodontium. *Int. Dent. J.*, **21**, 8.

Hamp, S. E., Nyman, S. and Lindhe, J. (1975). Periodontal treatment of multirooted teeth. Results after five years. *J. Clin. Periodont.*, **2**, 126.

Heaney, T. G. (1974). A reappraisal of environment, function and gingival specificity. *J. Periodontol.*, **45**, 695.

Hecht, A. and App, G. R. (1974). Blood volume lost during gingivectomy using two different anaesthetic techniques. *J. Periodontol.*, **45**, 9.

Helderman, W. H. V. P. and Hoogeveen, C. J. C. M. (1976). Bacterial enzymes and viable counts in crevices of non-inflamed and inflamed gingiva. *J. Periodont. Res.*, **11**, 25.

Horton, J. E., Leiken, S. and Oppenheim, J. J. (1972). Human lymphoproliferative reaction to saliva and dental plaque deposits. In vitro correlation with periodontal disease. *J. Periodontol.*, **43**, 522.

Hugoson, A. (1970). Gingival inflammation and female sex hormones. *J. Periodont. Res.*, Supplement 5.

Ivanyi, L. and Lehner, T. (1970). Stimulation of lymphocyte transformation by bacterial antigen in patients with periodontal disease. *Arch. Oral Biol.*, **15**, 1089.

Jandinski, J. J. and Shklar, G. (1976). Lichen planus of the gingiva. *J. Periodontol.*, **47**, 724.

Jenkins, G. N. (1970). *The physiology of the mouth*. Oxford: Blackwell Scientific Publications.

Johnson, R. H. (1976). Basic flap management. *Dent. Clin. N. Amer.*, **20**, 3, Jan.

Karring, T., Cumming, B. R., Oliver, R. C. and Löe, H. (1975). The origin of granulation tissue and its impact on postoperative results of muco-gingival surgery. *J. Periodontol.*, **46**, 577.

Kaslick, R. S., Chasens, A. I., Tuckman, M. A. and Kaufman, B. (1971). Investigation of periodontosis with periodontitis. *J. Periodontol.*, **42**, 420.

Kenny, E. B., Kraal, J. H., Saxe, S. R. and Jones, J. (1977). The effect of cigarette smoke on human oral polymorphonuclear leucocytes. *J. Periodont. Res.*, **12**, 227.

Krasse, B. and Egelberg, J. (1962). The relative proportions of sodium, potassium, and calcium in gingival pocket fluid. *Acta Odontol. Scand.*, **20**, 143.

Lang, N. P. and Löe, H. (1972). The relationship between width of keratinized gingiva and gingival health. *J. Periodontol.*, **43**, 623.

Lehner, T., Wilton, J. M. A., Ivanyi, L. and Manson, J. D. (1974). Immunological aspects of juvenile periodontitis (periodontosis). *J. Periodont. Res.*, **9**, 261.

Lennon, M. A. and Davies, R. M. (1974). Prevalence and distribution of alveolar bone loss in a population of 15-year-old schoolchildren. *J. Clin. Periodont.*, **1**, 175.

Lindhe, J. and Björn, H. (1967). Influence of hormonal contraceptives on the gingiva of women. *J. Periodont. Res.*, **2**, 1.

Lindhe, J., Hamp, S-E. and Löe, H. (1975). Plaque-induced periodontal disease in beagle dogs – a four-year clinical, roentgenographical and histometric study. *J. Periodont. Res.*, **10**, 243.

Lindhe, J. and Svanberg, G. (1974). Influence of trauma from occlusion on progression of experimental periodontitis in the beagle dog. *J. Clin. Periodont.*, **1**, 3.

Listgarten, M. (1972). Gingival epithelium. *Oral Sciences Review 1*, Copenhagen: Munksgaard.

Listgarten, M. A., Mayo, H. E. and Tremblay, R. (1975). Development of dental plaque on epoxy resin crowns in man. *J. Periodontol.*, **46**, 10.

Löe, H. and Holm-Pedersen, P. H. (1965). Absence and presence of fluid from normal and inflamed gingivae. *Periodontics*, **3**, 171.

Löe H. and Rindom Schiøtt, C. (1970). The effect of mouth rinses and topical application of chlorhexidine on the development of dental plaque and gingivitis in man. *J. Periodont. Res.*, **5**, 79.

Löe, H. and Silness, J. (1963). Periodontal disease in pregnancy I. *Acta Odontol. Scand.*, **21**, 533.

Löe, H., Theilade, E. and Jenkins, S. B. (1965). Experimental gingivitis in man. *J. Periodontol.*, **36**, 177.

Mackler, S. B. and Crawford, J. J. (1973). Plaque development and gingivitis in the primary dentition. *J. Periodontol.*, **44**, 18.

Mackler, B. F., Frostad, K. B., Robertson, P. B. and Levy, B. M. (1977). Immunoglobulin bearing lymphocytes and plasma cells in human periodontal disease. *J. Periodont. Res.*, **12**, 37.

Melcher, A. H. and Eastoe, J. E. (1969). *Biology of the periodontium*. London, New York: Academic Press.

Miyasato, M. C. (1975). The periodontal abscess. *Periodontal Abstracts*, **23**, 53.

Miyasato, M., Crigger, M. and Egelberg, J. (1977). Gingival condition in areas of minimal and appreciable width of keratinized gingiva. *J. Clin. Periodont.*, **4**, 200.

Mühlemann, H. R. (1958). Gingivitis in Zurich schoolchildren. *Helv. Odont. Acta*, **2**, 3.

Newcombe, G. M. and Waite, I. M. (1972). The effectiveness of two local analgesic preparations in reducing haemorrhage during periodontal surgery. *J. Dent.*, **1**, 37.

Polson, A. M., Meitner, S. W. and Zander, H. A. (1976). Trauma and progression of marginal periodontitis in squirrel monkeys. *J. Periodont. Res.*, **11**, 279.

Poulton, D. R. and Aaronson, S. A. (1961). The relationship between occlusion and periodontal disease. *Am. J. Orthodont.*, **47**, 690.

Ramfjord, S. P., Nissle, R. R., Shick, R. A. and Cooper, H. (1968). Subgingival curettage versus surgical elimination of periodontal pockets. *J. Periodontol.*, **39**, 167.

Ranney, R. R. (1970). Specific antibody in gingiva and submandibular nodes of monkeys with allergic periodontal disease. *J. Periodont. Res.*, **5**, 1.

Ruggerio, A. C. (1975). Intravenous sedation of the periodontal surgical patient. *J. Periodontol.*, **46**, 319.

Russell, A. L. (1956). A system of classification and scoring for prevalence surveys of periodontal disease. *J. Dent. Res.*, **36**, 922.

Russell, A. L., Leatherwood, E. C., Consolazio, C. F. and Reen, R. V. (1965). Periodontal disease and nutrition in South Vietnam. *J. Dent. Res.*, **44**, 775.

Saxén, L., Aula, S. and Westermarck, T. (1977). Periodontal disease associated with Down's syndrome: an orthopantomographic evaluation. *J. Periodontol.*, **48**, 337.

Schwartz, J., Stinson, F. L. and Parker, R. B. (1972). The passage of tritiated bacterial endotoxin across intact gingival crevicular epithelium. *J. Periodontol.*, **43**, 270.

Shane, S. M. E. (1975). *Principles of sedation and general anaesthesia in dentistry*. Illinois: Thomas Publishers.

Sheiham, A. (1971). Periodontal disease and oral cleanliness in tobacco smokers. *J. Periodontol.*, **42**, 259.

Silness, J. and Löe, H. (1964). Periodontal disease in pregnancy II. *Acta Odontol. Scand.*, **22**, 121.

Simon, B. I., Goldman, H. M., Ruben, M. P., Broitman, S. and Baker, E. (1972). The rôle of endotoxin in periodontal disease IV. *J. Peridontol.*, **43**, 468.

Sims, W. (1976). Serum hepatitis and the dental surgeon. *J. Dent.*, **4**, 151.

Smith, F. N. and Lang, N. P. (1977). Lymphocyte blastogenesis to plaque antigens in human periodontal disease II: the relationship to clinical parameters. *J. Periodont. Res.*, **12**, 310.

Smukler, H. (1976). Laterally positioned mucoperiosteal grafts in the treatment of denuded roots. *J. Periodontol.*, **47**, 590.

Stahl, S. S., Slavkin, H. C., Yamada, L. and Levine, S. (1972). Speculations about gingival repair. *J. Periodontol.*, **43**, 395.

Stone, S., Ramfjord, S. P. and Waldron, J. (1965). Scaling and gingival curettage. A radioautographic study. *J. Periodontol.*, **37**, 415.

Strahan, J. D., Bashaarat, A. and Greenslade, R. N. (1977). Control of plaque by non chemical means. *J. Clin. Periodont.*, **4**, 513.

Strahan, J. D. and Glenwright, H. D. (1967). Pain experience in periodontal surgery. *J. Periodont. Res.*, **1**, 163.

Sugarman, M. M. (1970). In our opinion: occlusion. *J. Periodontol.*, **41**, 536.

Sullivan, H. C. and Atkins, J. H. (1968). Free autogenous gingival grafts: principles of successful grafting. *Periodontics*, **6**, 121.

Suomi, J. D., Greene, J. C., Vermillion, J. R., Chang, J. J. and Leatherwood, E. C. (1969). The effect of controlled oral hygiene on the progression of periodontal disease. *J. Periodontol.*, **40**, 416.

Suppipat, N. (1974). Ultrasonics in periodontics. *J. Clin. Periodont.*, **1**, 206.

Sutcliffe, P. (1972). A longitudinal study of gingivitis and puberty. *J. Periodont. Res.*, **7**, 52.

Svanberg, G. (1974). Influence of trauma from occlusion on the periodontium of dogs with normal or inflamed gingiva. *Odont. Revy.*, **25**, 165.

Svanberg, G. and Lindhe, J. (1974). Vascular reactions in the periodontal ligament incident to trauma from occlusion. *J. Clin. Periodont.*, **1**, 58.

Taichman, N. S. (1970). Mediation of inflammation by the polymorphonuclear leucocyte as a sequela of immune reactions. *J. Periodontol.*, **41**, 228.

Taichman, N. S. (1974). Some perspectives on the pathogenesis of periodontal disease. *J. Periodontol.*, **45**, 361.

Waite, I. M. (1975). The present status of the gingivectomy procedure. *J. Clin. Periodont.*, **2**, 241.

Ward, V. J. (1974). A clinical assessment of the use of the free gingival graft for correcting localised recession associated with frenal pull. *J. Periodont. Res.*, **45**, 78.

Weissman, B. (1965). A nonparallel universal horizontal pin splint. *J. Prosth. Dent.*, **15**, 339.

Wise, M. D. (1977). Occlusion and restorative dentistry. *Brit. Dent. J.*, **143**, 45.

Wood, D. L., Hoag, P. M., Donnenfield, O. W. and Rosenfeld, L. D. (1972). Alveolar crest reduction following full and partial thickness flaps. *J. Periodontol.*, **43**, 141.

Zachrisson, B. W. and Alnaes, L. (1973). Periodontal condition in orthodontically treated and untreated individuals I. *Angle Orthodont.*, **43**, 402.

Zachrisson, B. W. and Alnaes, L. (1974). Periodontal condition in orthodontically treated and untreated individuals II. *Angle Orthodont.*, **44**, 48.

Zachrisson, S. and Zachrisson, B. W. (1972). Gingival condition associated with orthodontic treatment. *Angle Orthodont.*, **42**, 26.

Index

All references are to page numbers.

A

Abscess, periodontal 37, 91
Acrylic veneer 109
Acute necrotising ulcerative gingivitis 36
Acute non-specific gingivitis 39
Acute periapical abscess 39
Acute periodontal abscess 37, 91
Adjustment, occlusal 96–101
Aetiology 15–22
Age, influence on periodontal disease 23, 24
Agranulocytosis 26
Alveolar bone 9
Alveolar mucosa 11
Amalgam tattoo 35
Antibodies 17
Antigens 17, 18
Aphthous ulceration 32
Apically repositioned flap 68
Assessment chart 41, 118, 120

B

Bass technique 45
Bite guard 102
Blood dyscrasias 26
Blood supply, gingiva 9
– periodontium 9
Bone, alveolar 9
– defects 72, 128, 129
– grafts 72–75
– regeneration 71, 72, 110
– rôle of extraction 77
Bridgework, rôle of 77
Bruxism 96, 99

C

Calculus, formation of 21
Calculus probe 51
Case history 40
Cellular (delayed) immune
    reaction 18, 28, 114
Chemical injury 32
Chisel scaler 53
Chlorhexidine 49
– staining 49
Combined periodontal and endodontic
    lesions 110, 111
Complement 17, 114
Congenital defects 14, 28, 29, 114
Conservative dentistry 21, 106, 107, 113
Coronally repositioned flap 87
Curettage, subgingival 55–57
Curette 52, 56, 64

D

Dehiscence 9
Dental plaque, see Plaque
Dentogingival junction 10, 11
Desquamative gingivitis 34
Deviation, mandibular 95, 97
Diabetes 27
Diagnosis 40–43
Diastema 81, 94
Disclosing of plaque 48
Displacement dressings 54
Down's syndrome 29
Dressing, post-surgical 62, 66, 124
– displacement 54
Drugs 26, 114
– post-operative 122
Drug therapy 33, 37, 38

E

Education of patient 44
Elastic fibres 11
Electric toothbrush 48
Endodontic implant 105
Endodontic therapy 76, 110, 111
Enzymes 17, 18
Epidemiology 23–25, 115
Extraction, rôle of 77

F

Fenestration 9
Fibromatosis gingivae 14
Floss 46, 47
Free-end saddle prostheses 113
Free gingiva 11
Frenectomy 78, 80
Frenum 13, 80, 81
Fibrous epulis 30
Furcation involvement 76, 110

G

Geographic distribution of periodontal disease 25
Giant cell granuloma 31
Gingivae, direct trauma to 13, 86, 91
Gingival enlargements 30
Gingival epithelium 10, 11, 132
Gingival fibres 10
Gingival fluid 16, 114
Gingival graft 82–87
Gingival hyperplasia 14, 26, 55, 58
Gingival pigmentation 11, 34, 35
Gingival recession 9, 13, 85, 87, 88
Gingival sulcus 10, 11
Gingival width 12, 13, 82
Gingivectomy 58–62, 108, 109
– healing 131
Gingivitis, acute 32, 33, 36–39
– aetiology 15–23
– blood dyscrasias 26, 114
– drugs 26, 32, 34, 114
– hormonal 23, 27, 31, 114
– hyperplastic 26, 30, 31

H

Habits 94, 96
Heavy metals, pigmentation 34
Herpes simplex 33
Histopathology, localised gingival enlargements 32
– periodontal disease 17
Hormonal changes 23, 27, 31, 114
Host response 17–20, 26–29, 114
Humoral immune response 17, 114
Hydantoin 26

I

Immunology 16, 17, 114
Incision, curettage 56, 57
– frenectomy 78, 79
– gingivectomy 58, 60
– inverse bevel flap 63, 64
– laterally repositioned flap 88, 89
Increased overbite 13, 86, 91
Increased overjet 22, 90
Indications, flap procedure 63
– gingival graft 82
– gingivectomy 58
– laterally repositioned flap 88
– occlusal adjustment 96
– osseous surgery 69
Indices 23, 115
Induction of keratinization 132
Inflammation, see Gingivitis and Periodontal disease
Infra-bony defect 38, 71–75, 96, 128, 129
Instruction in plaque control 45
Instruments, surgical 126, 127
Interdental cleaning 46–48
Interdental papillae 11, 12
Interdental sticks 47
Interproximal brush 48, 76
Inverse bevel flap 38, 63–68, 112, 113, 130, 132

J

Junctional epithelium 10
Juvenile periodontitis 28

K

Keratinization, induction of 132

L

Labial veneer 109
Laterally repositioned flap 88, 89
Lichen planus 34
Lip posture 22, 90, 94
Lip seal, lack of 22, 90
Local analgesia 59, 125
Lymphocyte transformation 18, 114
Lysosomal granules 18

M

Malocclusion 90, 91
Management of patient 122–124
Medical history 40
Metabolites from plaque 17, 114
Microorganisms 15, 16, 36, 38
Migration of teeth 94, 112
Mobility, assessment 42
Motivation of patient 44
Mucogingival junction 11, 12
Mucosa, alveolar 11
Mucosal lesions 32–35

N

Nutrition 25

O

Occlusal adjustment 96–101
Occlusal analysis 96–101
Occlusal trauma 92, 93, 96
Odontoplasty 76
Oral hygiene, see Plaque control
Orthodontic treatment 81, 91, 112, 113
Osseous defects 38, 71–75, 96, 128, 129
Osseous surgery 69–75
Overbite, increased 13, 86, 91
Overjet, increased 22, 90

P

Palatal groove 14
Papilloma 32
Papillon Lefèvre syndrome 28
Patient management 122–124
Pellicle 15
Periapical abscess 39, 110, 111
Periodontal abscess 37–39, 91
Periodontal chart 41, 118, 120
Periodontal disease, aetiology 15–22
– children 23, 24, 27, 28
– geographical distribution 25
– host response 17, 19, 26–29, 114
– influence of occlusion 90–95
– influence of orthodontic treatment 91
– nutrition 25
– oral hygiene 24
– race 25
– socio-economic factors 25
Periodontal dressing 54, 62, 66, 79, 84, 124
Periodontal examination 40–43, 116–120
Periodontal indices 23, 115
Periodontal ligament 9
Periodontal pocket, measurement 41, 55
Periodontal surgery, instrumentation 126, 127
– marking of pockets 59
– rationale 55
Periodontal therapy, rôle of extraction 77
Periodontitis, see Periodontal disease
Periodontosis 28
Periosteal retention 64
Pigmentation 11, 34, 35
Plaque 15–22
– control 44–49, 121
– disclosing 44, 48
– formation 15
– protective mechanism 114
– relation to inflammation 21, 24
– retention 21, 22, 91, 107–109
– structure 15, 16
Plasma cells 17, 18
Pockets, infra-bony 38, 71–75, 96, 128, 129
– soft tissue 14, 20, 41, 54, 55, 58, 63
Polishing of teeth 53
Polymorphs 17, 18
Post operative care 122
Pregnancy 27, 31

Primary trauma 92
Probe, calculus 51
– pocket measuring 10, 55
Prostheses, plaque retention 21, 108, 109
Prosthetic dentistry 108, 109
Protective mechanisms against plaque 114
Puberty 23, 27
Pyogenic granuloma 30, 31

R

Race, periodontal disease 25
Radiography 42, 43
Rationale for periodontal surgery 55
Recession, treatment of 82–89
Regeneration, bone 71, 72, 110
Reinforcement of plaque control 48
Restorations, plaque retention 21, 107, 108
– relation to gingival margin 21, 106, 107
Restorative dentistry 21, 107–113
Retention, of plaque 21, 22, 91, 107–109
– post-orthodontic treatment 102, 113
Root amputation 76

S

Scaling 50–52
Secondary trauma 93, 96
Sequence of treatment 112, 121
Sex, influence on periodontal disease 23
Socio-economic factors, influence on periodontal disease 25
Soft tissue forces 94
Splints 77, 102–106, 113
Subgingival curettage 55–57
Sulcular epithelium 10, 17
Sulcus contents 16
Sutures 65, 74, 79, 83, 89, 130
Systemic factors 26–29, 31, 114

T

Tissue response 17–20
Tobacco smoking 22, 37
Toothbrushing 45, 46
– trauma from 13
Tooth deposits 15, 16
– recording 42, 115
Tooth stains, chlorhexidine 49
Toxins 17, 114
Trauma, direct gingival 13, 86, 91
– from occlusion 92, 93, 96
– primary occlusal 92
– secondary occlusal 93, 96
Treatment planning 112, 122–124
Trephine 73
Tuberosity 14
– management of 68

U

Ulcers, aphthous 32
Ultrasonic scaler 50

V

Vincent's gingivitis 36

W

Water jet instrument 49
Width of gingivae 12, 13, 82
Wound healing 131, 132